Mosby's

HANDBOOK OF
DRUG-HERB AND
DRUG-SUPPLEMENT
INTERACTIONS

Richard Harkness, Pharm, CDM, FASCP
President, TPC Consultants
Ocean Springs, Mississippi

Steven Bratman, MD
Consulting Editor of Complementary
and Alternative Medicine for HealthGate Data Corp.
Fort Collins, Colorado

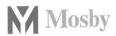 Mosby

An Affiliate of Elsevier Science
St. Louis   London   Philadelphia   Sydney   Toronto

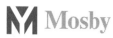
Mosby

An Affiliate of Elsevier Science

11830 Westline Industrial Drive
St. Louis, Missouri 63146

MOSBY'S HANDBOOK OF DRUG-HERB
AND DRUG-SUPPLEMENT INTERACTIONS   ISBN 0-323-02014-3
Copyright © 2003, Mosby, Inc. All rights reserved.

NOTICE

Knowledge regarding the proper use of herbs and supplements is ever
changing. Standard safety precautions must be followed, but as new research and clinical experience broaden our understanding, changes in
use may become necessary or appropriate. Readers are advised to check
the most current product information provided by the manufacturer of
each product to be administered to verify the recommended dose, the
method and duration of administration, and contraindications. It is the
responsibility of the treating licensed practitioner, relying on experience and knowledge of the patient, to determine dosages and the best
treatment for each individual patient.

This publication is not intended as a substitute for medical therapy nor
as a manual for self-treatment. Readers should seek professional advice
for any specific medical problems.

Neither the Publisher nor the author assumes any liability for any injury
and/or damage to persons or property arising from this publication.

International Standard Book Number 0-323-02014-3

Publishing Director: Linda L. Duncan
Acquisitions Editor: Kellie F. White
Associate Developmental Editor: Jennifer L. Watrous
Publishing Services Manager: Linda McKinley
Project Manager: Judy Ahlers
Designer: Julia Dummitt
Cover Art: Sheilah Barrett

TG/QWF

Printed in the United States of America

9   8   7   6   5   4   3   2   1

INTRODUCTION

Natural medicine, including herbs, vitamins, minerals, and various other supplements, has surged to enormous popularity in recent years. In the companion volume to this one, *Mosby's Handbook of Herbs and Supplements and Their Therapeutic Uses*, we discuss the clinical evidence for and against the use of these treatments, as well as dosage and safety issues. In this book, *Mosby's Handbook of Drug-Herb and Drug-Supplement Interactions*, we focus entirely on the most important safety issue with such "natural therapies": drug interactions.

As with drug-drug interactions, drug-herb and drug-supplement interactions can present significant health risks. All the same categories of interaction exist, including potentiation of drug effects, interference with drug action, alteration of drug absorption and metabolism, and amplification of risks and side effects. Some of these interactions may be life-threatening if not recognized, whereas others may present no more than an insignificant or theoretical risk.

Like standard works on drug-drug interactions, *Mosby's Handbook of Drug-Herb and Drug-Supplement Interactions* is organized by interaction exemplar. Potential interactions involving related agents are also listed. To access this information most effectively, it is best to look up drugs, herbs, or natural supplements in the index and refer to the page numbers provided to review known or suspected interactions.

Each interaction is rated according to the following numerical key:

Rating	Description
1	Significant interaction
2	Possibly significant interaction
3	Interaction of relatively little significance
4	Reported interaction that does not, in fact, exist or is insignificant

Readers will next find a brief summary of the interaction, followed by analysis of the evidence on which the presumed interaction is based. Each article concludes with suggestions for medical management.

Note: Patients frequently do not spontaneously disclose what over-the-counter supplements they may be using. The physician must ask direct, open-ended questions to identify such usage. A strong argument can be made for querying about this at each patient encounter. This applies to all demographics, as usage of "alternative medicine" has begun to pervade society at large. Timely questioning and usage of *Mosby's Handbook of Drug-Herb and Drug-Supplement Interactions* may prevent significant patient harm.

Steven Bratman, MD
Consulting Editor
COMPLEMENTARY AND ALTERNATIVE MEDICINE
FOR HEALTHGATE DATA CORP.

CONTENTS

Mosby's

HANDBOOK OF
DRUG-HERB AND
DRUG-SUPPLEMENT
INTERACTIONS

INTERACTIONS

5-HTP—
LEVODOPA/CARBIDOPA

Rating 2

Interaction Summary

Taking 5-HTP (5-hydroxytryptophan) and carbidopa together might cause a scleroderma-like syndrome.

Discussion

Syndromes resembling scleroderma have been reported in individuals with abnormalities of tryptophan metabolism.[1,2] The development of this condition is believed to involve two factors: elevated plasma serotonin and the abnormality associated with elevated kynurenine.[2]

Tryptophan is a precursor of 5-hydroxytryptophan (5-HTP), which in turn is converted into serotonin. The combination of 5-HTP and carbidopa, sometimes used as treatment for intention myoclonus, has also been associated with such syndromes.[1,2]

One case report suggested that carbidopa unmasked an abnormality in one of the enzymes that catabolize kynurenine, an intermediate compound in tryptophan metabolism, leading to elevated levels of this metabolite.[2] Individuals vulnerable to this interaction may be those with the enzyme abnormality. Withdrawal of the 5-HTP resulted in a decline in plasma kynurenine,

---

Rating Scale:
(1) Significant interaction
(2) Possibly significant interaction
(3) Interaction of relatively little significance
(4) Reported interaction that does not, in fact, exist or is insignificant

3

and initiation of oral vitamin B_6 at 100 mg daily was accompanied by continued clinical improvement of the scleroderma.

Management Suggestions

Patients taking carbidopa should avoid supplemental 5-HTP.

ACE INHIBITORS—IRON

RELATED DRUGS

Benazepril
Captopril
Enalapril
Fosinopril

Lisinopril
Quinapril
Ramipril

RELATED SUPPLEMENTS

Ferrous fumarate
Ferrous gluconate

Ferrous sulfate
Iron polysaccharide

Interaction Summary

Iron supplements can interfere with the absorption of captopril and perhaps other ACE inhibitors. Conversely, iron absorption also may be impaired.

Discussion

Captopril appears to bind with iron to form a nonabsorbable complex.[1] This may impair absorption of both the drug and the nutrient.

Rating Scale:
(1) Significant interaction
(2) Possibly significant interaction
(3) Interaction of relatively little significance
(4) Reported interaction that does not, in fact, exist or is insignificant

Management Suggestions

To minimize any potential problems, administer iron supplements (if needed) and ACE inhibitors 2 to 3 hours apart.

ACE INHIBITORS—POTASSIUM

RELATED DRUGS

Benazepril   Lisinopril

Captopril   Quinapril

Enalapril   Ramipril

Fosinopril

Interaction Summary

Combining potassium with captopril or other ACE inhibitors may cause hyperkalemia.

Discussion

ACE inhibitor–induced reduction of angiotensin II levels diminishes aldosterone secretion, causing potassium retention. Patients on ACE inhibitors may not realize that ingesting relatively high levels of potassium from diet or supplements can raise potassium levels too high, and physicians may not be aware that their patients are receiving additional potassium.

Of 386 patients identified with hyperkalemia in one institution, 114 were taking an ACE inhibitor.[1] Of the patients consenting to an interview, 72% were found to be consuming moderate to high amounts of potassium in their diets.

Rating Scale:

(1) Significant interaction

(2) Possibly significant interaction

(3) Interaction of relatively little significance

(4) Reported interaction that does not, in fact, exist or is insignificant

Case reports have found that serum potassium levels moved from normal to high in patients taking captopril along with potassium supplementation or a potassium-sparing diuretic.[2,3,4] A patient on lisinopril and consuming a potassium-rich diet was found to have a serum potassium level of 9.7 mEq/L.[5]

Symptoms of hyperkalemia include cardiac arrhythmias, muscle weakness, nausea, vomiting, irritability, and diarrhea.

Management Suggestions

Question patients to determine whether they might be ingesting a high-potassium diet or taking a potassium supplement, salt substitute containing potassium, or potassium-sparing diuretic. Monitor serum potassium concentrations and adjust potassium intake as needed.

ACETAMINOPHEN—VITAMIN C

Interaction Summary

Very high doses of vitamin C (3 g daily) might impair metabolism of acetaminophen, potentially increasing serum levels.

Discussion

In one small 1976 study, 5 volunteer subjects took 3000 mg of vitamin C 1.5 hours after taking 1000 mg of acetaminophen.[1] The net effect was a modest increase in the apparent half-life of acetaminophen, from 2.3 to 3.1 hours.

Ascorbic acid competitively inhibits the hepatic metabolism of acetaminophen to the inactive sulfate metabolite, thus decreasing the excretion rate of this fraction.[1] However, the liver metabolizes most acetaminophen to the inactive glucuronide metabolite. If metabolism to the sulfate metabolite is impaired, a compensatory mechanism might increase the fractions of acetaminophen glucuronide as well as unchanged drug excreted. Although these two processes partially offset each other, it is possible that the net effect will be reduced acetaminophen excretion.

This interaction probably has little clinical significance when acetaminophen is taken in single therapeutic doses for pain and fever. However, it could potentially present a problem with

---

Rating Scale:

(1) Significant interaction

(2) Possibly significant interaction

(3) Interaction of relatively little significance

(4) Reported interaction that does not, in fact, exist or is insignificant

long-term acetaminophen use or in individuals with impaired hepatic or renal function.

Management Suggestions

Individuals on chronic acetaminophen therapy may be advised to avoid high-dose vitamin C supplementation. This interaction may be of particular importance for those with renal or hepatic disease.

ALPRAZOLAM—KAVA

Rating 2

RELATED DRUGS

Chlordiazepoxide	Lorazepam
Clorazepate	Oxazepam
Diazepam	Prazepam

Interaction Summary

Concomitant use may result in central nervous system depression with accompanying sedation and drowsiness.

Discussion

In a single case report, a 54-year-old man was hospitalized for lethargy and disorientation following 3 days of kava intake concomitantly with alprazolam.[1] His other medications included cimetidine and terazosin in undisclosed amounts. Cimetidine, a cytochrome p450 inhibitor, can inhibit alprazolam metabolism resulting in sedation and lethargy, but this had not been experienced previously in the patient. The temporal relationship strongly suggests that the addition of kava adversely affected the patient's sensorium.

It has been suggested that the kavapyrones present in kava preparations are responsible for such events. In a rat study of [^{3}H]-muscimol binding, regional differences in GABA$_A$-receptor

---

Rating Scale:
(1) Significant interaction
(2) Possibly significant interaction
(3) Interaction of relatively little significance
(4) Reported interaction that does not, in fact, exist or is insignificant

binding were found with preferential binding in the hippocampus and less in the amygdala and medulla oblongata.[2] A concentration-dependent increase of [^{3}H]-GABA binding of 358% to the GABA$_A$ receptor was caused by a lipophilic kava extract. Further analysis revealed that the kavapyrones' effect was due to an increase in the number of binding sites (B$_{max}$) rather than a change in receptor affinity.[2]

Additive effects on [^{3}H]-muscimol binding were observed when the kavapyrones were combined with pentobarbital. However, in another study, kavapyrones were found to exert a weak effect on benzodiazepine binding in vitro.[3] When compared to controls, the kavapyrones dihydromethysticin and tetrahydroyangonin at a concentration of 1 mM bound to the receptors at 74% ± 2% ($P < 0.01$) and 78% ± 3% ($P < 0.001$), respectively. Perhaps key to this study observation was that the tissue originated from the forebrain, recalling the regional differences in binding noted by Jussofie et al.[2] Davies et al. concluded that lipophilic kavapyrones were integrated into the lipid membranes, leading to a nonspecific modification of the GABA$_A$ receptor conformation.[3]

More modest effects were noted in another study, with the maximal increase of the specific [^{3}H]-BMC binding of 18% to 28% using 0.1 μmol of (+)-kavain, (+)-methysticin, (+)-dihydromethysticin, and 10 μmol of (+)-dihydrokavain.[4] Dopaminergic and serotonergic receptors were unaffected in rat studies using oral doses of 100 mg (+)-dihydromethysticin/kg body weight, as revealed by striatal and cortical tissue concentrations.[5]

Thus the effect of kavapyrones apparently is dose dependent and site specific. Coupled with the clinical observation of Almeida and Grimsley,[1] concomitant use with benzodiazepines or other agents affecting GABA receptors appears to be ill-advised.

Management Suggestions

Concomitant use of kava with alprazolam or any of the other benzodiazepines is not recommended. For patients insisting on combining the two, counsel should include a description of possible central nervous system side effects, such as sedation, grogginess, and disorientation. Furthermore, these patients should be advised to avoid activity requiring mental alertness.

ALUMINUM HYDROXIDE— CALCIUM CITRATE

Rating 3

Interaction Summary

Concerns have been raised that the aluminum in aluminum-containing antacids may present a health risk. There is evidence that calcium citrate and other citrates may increase the absorption of aluminum from antacids as well as dietary sources, thus increasing the risk.

Discussion

In a 3-day study of 10 normal volunteers, the combination of calcium citrate and aluminum hydroxide gel (an antacid) caused a significant increase in the absorption of aluminum compared to aluminum hydroxide gel alone.[1] In contrast, calcium acetate did not produce a significant change in aluminum absorption compared to aluminum hydroxide gel alone. Aluminum absorption was determined by measuring aluminum plasma levels and urine excretion levels.

Another study of 30 women taking calcium citrate supplements to prevent osteoporosis found increased aluminum absorption from dietary sources, which include baking powder and nondairy creamers (other aluminum-containing products were prohibited during this study).[2] This increased dietary aluminum absorption may not be a significant problem in individuals with

---

Rating Scale:

(1) Significant interaction

(2) Possibly significant interaction

(3) Interaction of relatively little significance

(4) Reported interaction that does not, in fact, exist or is insignificant

normal kidney function, because urinary excretion of aluminum increases as absorption increases. However, individuals with impaired kidney function may be at increased risk.

Studies of other citrates (e.g., sodium citrate) have found effects on aluminum absorption similar to those associated with calcium citrate.[3,4] Experimental studies in rats suggest that citrate may increase the gastrointestinal absorption of aluminum by enhancing its solubility.[5]

Management Suggestions

To help minimize potential toxicity, administering calcium citrate supplements apart from aluminum-containing antacids and meals is advisable.

When treating individuals with hyperphosphatemia, calcium acetate may be preferable to calcium citrate when administered with aluminum hydroxide gel to bind phosphate, especially in chronic renal failure patients.

AMIODARONE—CHAPARRAL

Rating 2

RELATED DRUGS

Androgenic steroids	Niacin
Fibric acids	Statin drugs
Hepatotoxic drugs	Tacrine
Ketoconazole	

Interaction Summary

Reports suggest that chaparral may hasten the onset and worsen the severity of the hepatotoxicity of known hepatotoxic drugs, such as amiodarone, androgenic steroids, fibric acids, ketoconazole, niacin, statin drugs, and tacrine. However, this suggestion remains controversial.

Discussion

Toxic hepatitis and subacute hepatic necrosis have been reported among individuals using chaparral, with some cases of sufficient severity to require liver transplantation.[1-5] In a review of 18 cases of chaparral-induced illnesses reported to the Food and Drug Administration (FDA) between 1992 and 1994, 13 had evidence of hepatotoxicity, such as jaundice and marked increase in serum liver chemistries, with onset noted within 3 to 52 weeks after chaparral ingestion.[6] Symptoms resolved within 1 to 17 weeks after discontinuation. The authors noted that in 10 of these

---

Rating Scale:

(1) Significant interaction
(2) Possibly significant interaction

(3) Interaction of relatively little significance
(4) Reported interaction that does not, in fact, exist or is insignificant

cases the evidence was compelling enough to clearly implicate chaparral as the cause.

Furthermore, nordihydroguaiaretic acid, a lignan component of chaparral, has been shown to inhibit cytochrome p450–mediated monooxygenase activity in rat microsomes.[7] In human and rat studies, nordihydroguaiaretic acid has been found to inhibit 5-lipoxygenase.[7,8] This may have implications for drugs metabolized by similar metabolic pathways.

Given these data, prudence would dictate avoiding concomitant use of chaparral and hepatotoxic drugs, such as amiodarone, androgenic steroids, and ketoconazole. A complete list of hepatotoxic drugs can be found in Jim and Gee.[9]

Management Suggestions

If possible, avoid concomitant use of chaparral and any known hepatotoxins. If taken together, the onset and severity of hepatic injury may be hastened and worsened. If both agents must be taken together, obtain baseline liver function tests, and test liver function 6 weeks later, then every 3 months for the first year, and periodically thereafter.

ASPIRIN—FISH OIL

Interaction Summary

Fish oil, a source of omega-3 fatty acids, has eicosanoid-modifying effects. Early evidence suggested that fish oil might cause increased risk of bleeding complications. However, one study found no evidence of increased risk when fish oil was combined with aspirin.

Discussion

Contrary to early reports, accumulating evidence suggests that fish oil does increase risk of bleeding complications when taken by itself.[1]

In a double-blind trial designed to determine whether the use of fish oil can prevent restenosis after coronary angioplasty, 551 individuals were given corn oil placebo or high-dose fish oil (8 g/day of omega-3 fatty acids) for a period of 6 months postoperatively.[2] All participants concurrently received 325 mg/day aspirin. The results showed no increased risk of bleeding complications in the group receiving fish oil.

Management Suggestions

Based on current evidence, it appears that fish oil can be combined safely with aspirin therapy.

Rating Scale:
(1) Significant interaction
(2) Possibly significant interaction

(3) Interaction of relatively little significance
(4) Reported interaction that does not, in fact, exist or is insignificant

ASPIRIN—POLICOSANOL

Rating 2

RELATED DRUGS

NSAIDs
  Bromfenac
  Diclofenac
  Etodolac
  Fenoprofen
  Flurbiprofen
  Ibuprofen
  Indomethacin
  Ketoprofen
  Ketorolac
  Meclofenamate
  Mefenamic acid
  Nabumetone
  Naproxen
Oxaprozin
Piroxicam
Sulindac
Tolmetin
Other drugs
  Abciximab
  Anagrelide
  Cilostazol
  Clopidogrel
  Dipyridamole
  Eptifibatide
  Pentoxifylline
  Ticlopidine
  Tirofiban

OTHER POTENTIALLY IMPLICATED SUPPLEMENTS

Feverfew
Ginger
Saw palmetto
White willow

Rating Scale:
(1) Significant interaction
(2) Possibly significant interaction
(3) Interaction of relatively little significance
(4) Reported interaction that does not, in fact, exist or is insignificant

Interaction Summary

Policosanol has antiplatelet actions that might potentiate the anticoagulant effect of aspirin and other antiplatelet agents.

In one case report, use of the herb saw palmetto was associated with significantly increased bleeding time and intraoperative hemorrhage.[1]

White willow contains salicylates. Feverfew and ginger are known to affect platelet aggregation, although the clinical significance of these findings is unclear.

Discussion

Human trials have found that the supplement policosanol, used for hyperlipidemia, exhibits dose-dependent antiplatelet actions.[2,3] This effect is comparable to that of aspirin, and combined treatment produces an additive effect.[4]

A 30-day, double-blind, placebo-controlled trial of 27 individuals with hypercholesterolemia found that policosanol at 10 mg/day markedly reduced platelet aggregation induced by collagen, low-dose ADP, or arachidonic acid.[2]

A double-blind, placebo-controlled study of 37 healthy volunteers found evidence of a dose-dependent effect.[3] In this trial, participants received placebo or policosanol, 10 mg/day for 7 days, following a 7-day placebo washout period. For a subsequent 7 days the number of tablets was doubled, and then doubled again for a final 7 days. The results showed that antiplatelet effects in the treated group increased throughout the study, suggesting a dose-dependent relationship. However, a time effect cannot be ruled out.

A double-blind, placebo-controlled study of 43 healthy volunteers compared the effects of policosanol (20 mg/day), aspirin (100 mg/day), and combination therapy versus placebo.[4] The results showed that policosanol reduced ADP-induced platelet aggregation by 37%, epinephrine-induced aggregation by 21.9%, and collagen-induced aggregation by 40.5%. Aspirin reduced collagen-induced aggregation by 61.4% and epinephrine-induced aggregation by 21.9% but did not reduce ADP-induced aggregation. Combined therapy exhibited additive effects.

Management Suggestions

Concurrent use of policosanol and aspirin may warrant medical supervision.

ASPIRIN—VITAMIN E

RELATED DRUGS

NSAIDs
- Bromfenac
- Diclofenac
- Etodolac
- Fenoprofen
- Flurbiprofen
- Ibuprofen
- Indomethacin
- Ketoprofen
- Ketorolac
- Meclofenamate
- Mefenamic acid
- Nabumetone
- Naproxen
- Oxaprozin
- Piroxicam
- Sulindac
- Tolmetin

Other drugs
- Abciximab
- Anagrelide
- Cilostazol
- Clopidogrel
- Dipyridamole
- Eptifibatide
- Pentoxifylline
- Ticlopidine
- Tirofiban

OTHER POTENTIALLY IMPLICATED SUPPLEMENTS

Aortic glycosaminoglycans (GAGs)
Bromelain
Oligomeric proanthocyanidin complexes (OPCs)

Rating Scale:
(1) Significant interaction
(2) Possibly significant interaction
(3) Interaction of relatively little significance
(4) Reported interaction that does not, in fact, exist or is insignificant

Interaction Summary

Vitamin E appears to add to aspirin's antithrombotic effects, and the combination may be more effective than aspirin alone in preventing transient ischemic attacks (TIAs). However, it might also present an increased risk of hemorrhagic strokes and other abnormal bleeding episodes.

Discussion

Vitamin E has been shown to inhibit platelet aggregation in vitro.[1]

Liede et al.[2] studied vitamin E's effect on gingival bleeding in a random sample of 409 male smokers who had participated in the Alpha-Tocopherol, Beta-Carotene Cancer Prevention Study (ATBC study). Of these men, 191 had received alpha-tocopherol supplementation of 50 mg/day; 56 received aspirin (ASA); 30 received both; and 132 received neither. At the end of the ATBC study, gingival bleeding was found to be more common in those who had received alpha-tocopherol alone compared to nonusers ($P < 0.05$), whereas ASA alone increased bleeding only slightly. The highest incidence of gingival bleeding was among those taking alpha-tocopherol and ASA: 33.4% of probed sites bleeding versus 25.8% among subjects taking neither alpha-tocopherol nor ASA ($P < 0.001$). The daily dose of aspirin varied, but in each case exceeded 100 mg/day, a dose commonly used to prevent thrombosis. This study suggests that a relatively small daily dose of vitamin E could have a clinically important effect on coagulation, particularly with concurrent aspirin use.

A double-blind, randomized study in 100 patients with TIAs, minor strokes, or residual ischemic neurologic deficits found that a combination of vitamin E and aspirin significantly enhanced the efficacy of the preventive regimen.[3] There was a significant reduction in platelet adhesiveness in patients taking vitamin E (400 IU/day) plus aspirin (325 mg/day) compared with those taking aspirin alone.

In a study of 28,519 men, vitamin E supplementation at a dose of about 50 IU/day reduced the risk of ischemic stroke but was associated with an increased incidence of fatal hemorrhagic stroke.[4]

Management Suggestions

Concurrent use of vitamin E and aspirin may warrant medical supervision.

BETA-BLOCKERS—
CALCIUM

Rating 4

RELATED DRUGS

Acebutolol	Nadolol
Atenolol	Penbutolol
Betaxolol	Pindolol
Bisoprolol	Propranolol
Carteolol	Sotalol
Esmolol	Timolol
Metoprolol	

Interaction Summary

Calcium supplements may decrease blood levels of the beta-blocker atenolol and possibly other beta-blockers, although the clinical effects appear to be minimal after several doses.

Discussion

In a crossover study of six healthy subjects, coadministration of a calcium supplement with atenolol distinctly altered drug kinetics compared to atenolol administered alone.[1] Calcium, 500 mg (as the lactate, gluconate, and carbonate), given with atenolol, 100 mg, for 6 days decreased mean peak plasma levels (C_{max}) of atenolol by 51% and area under the plasma level–time

Rating Scale:
(1) Significant interaction
(2) Possibly significant interaction

(3) Interaction of relatively little significance
(4) Reported interaction that does not, in fact, exist or is insignificant

curve ($AUC_{0-\infty}$) by 32%. Twelve hours after a single dose of the atenolol-calcium combination, inhibition of exercise tachycardia was only 10% compared to 21% with atenolol alone. Atenolol plasma levels reached a mean value of 108 ng/ml 12 hours after coadministration with calcium compared to 190 ng/ml 12 hours after atenolol alone.

One mechanism for this interaction may involve impaired atenolol absorption due to complexing of the drug with calcium ions in the intestine, similar to the effect observed with calcium and tetracycline. Another possible mechanism is increased volume of distribution.

The change in atenolol levels appears to be short-lived. Elimination half-life ($t_{1/2}$) increased to 11 hours compared with 6.2 hours for atenolol alone. Over time, atenolol levels therefore rise. Atenolol C_{max} was lowered by only 21% after multiple oral doses of atenolol compared to 51% after the single dose. During a 4-week treatment of six hypertensive patients as part of the same study, blood pressure measurements for those taking the atenolol-calcium combination were similar to those taking atenolol alone, and no dosage adjustment was recommended. However, researchers recommended that patients with severe coronary artery disease be given twice the normal dose of atenolol on the first day of atenolol-calcium treatment.

Management Suggestions

No dosage adjustment appears necessary when atenolol is taken with calcium over the long term. As a precaution, however, giving patients with severe coronary artery disease twice the normal dose of atenolol on the first day of atenolol-calcium treatment may be advisable.

BIOTIN—CARBAMAZEPINE

Rating 3

RELATED DRUGS

Phenobarbital	Primidone
Phenytoin	Valproic acid

Interaction Summary

Carbamazepine may deplete biotin, possibly by competing with it for absorption in the intestine. It is not clear, however, whether this effect is harmful. Valproate may affect biotin to a lesser extent than other anticonvulsants.

Discussion

Plasma levels of biotin, an essential water-soluble B vitamin, were found to be substantially lower in 404 patients with epilepsy on long-term treatment with anticonvulsants compared to 112 untreated subjects serving as controls.[1] These lower biotin levels occurred with patients on monotherapy with phenytoin, carbamazepine, phenobarbital, or primidone (patients on monotherapy with sodium valproate, which differs chemically from the other anticonvulsants, had significantly higher biotin levels than those on one of the other anticonvulsants). Biotin was reduced more significantly than levels of other vitamins,

---

Rating Scale:
(1) Significant interaction
(2) Possibly significant interaction

(3) Interaction of relatively little significance
(4) Reported interaction that does not, in fact, exist or is insignificant

such as folate and vitamin D, known to be affected by anticonvulsant therapy. Additionally, the drug effect on biotin was dose dependent.

It is possible that lowered biotin levels could play a role in the mechanism of action of anticonvulsants. A reduction in biotin-dependent carboxylases could result in higher cerebral concentrations of free carbon dioxide, which would elevate the seizure threshold. However, this has not been proved.

An in vitro study may shed light on the manner in which anticonvulsants might lower biotin levels.[2] Examination of human intestinal tissue indicated that carbamazepine and primidone inhibit biotin transport in the intestine. This competitive inhibition occurred at the intestinal brush border membrane in a concentration-dependent manner.

Management Suggestions

Biotin supplementation may be advisable in patients on long-term anticonvulsant therapy. To avoid an absorptive interaction, administer a supplement 2 to 3 hours apart from the drug. Because it has been suggested that the action of anticonvulsant drugs may be at least in part related to their biotin-reducing effects, it may be desirable to administer enough biotin to prevent a deficiency, but not an excessive amount. The recommended adult daily value (DV) for biotin is 30 μg.

BROMOCRIPTINE— CHASTEBERRY

Rating 2

RELATED DRUGS

Amantadine
Chlorpromazine
Fluphenazine
Levodopa
Loxapine
Mesoridazine
Metoclopramide
Molindone
Pergolide
Perphenazine

Pimozide
Pramipexole
Prochlorperazine
Promazine
Ropinirole
Thioridazine
Thiothixene
Trifluoperazine
Triflupromazine

Interaction Summary

The ability of chasteberry to inhibit prolactin release may augment bromocriptine's prolactin-inhibitory effects. Similar interactions may be noted with other dopamine agonists, such as amantadine, levodopa, pergolide, pramipexole, and ropinirole.

In addition, dopamine antagonists may diminish chasteberry's effect (e.g., chlorpromazine, fluphenazine, loxapine, mesoridazine, metoclopramide, molindone, perphenazine, pimozide, prochlorperazine, promazine, thioridazine, thiothixene, trifluoperazine, and triflupromazine).

Rating Scale:
(1) Significant interaction
(2) Possibly significant interaction

(3) Interaction of relatively little significance
(4) Reported interaction that does not, in fact, exist or is insignificant

Discussion

Chasteberry is the dried ripe fruit of *Vitex agnus castus*. It is used for cyclic mastalgia, other premenstrual symptoms, irregularities of the menstrual cycle (specifically luteal phase defect), and infertility. Its active constituents are thought to be the iridoid glycosides, agnoside, and aucubin.

Dopamine agonist activity has been demonstrated in a rat pituitary cell culture model in which as little as 0.125 mg of chasteberry extract/ml significantly suppressed prolactin release.[1] The authors concluded that chasteberry binds to dopamine receptors (lactotropes) in the pituitary, resulting in inhibition of prolactin secretion. Because other neurotransmitters (e.g., GABA) can inhibit prolactin secretion, these same investigators tested chasteberry using the rat striatum domoic acid receptor assay, confirming that chasteberry's effect is mediated through dopamine.[1] Furthermore, chasteberry's effects are thought to be specific to the D_2 receptor.[2]

Human studies further validate this explanation. A 3-month, double-blind, placebo-controlled study of 52 women with luteal phase defects (shortened luteal phase with deficient progesterone synthesis) found that chasteberry treatment produced significant reduction in prolactin release and normalization of the luteal phase interval.[3] Hence, chasteberry apparently exerts a clinically significant effect on prolactin levels, and thus the potential exists for it to interact with drugs known to affect prolactin (e.g., dopamine agonists and antagonists).

Management Suggestions

Because human and animal studies suggest that chasteberry inhibits prolactin release, concomitant use with bromocriptine or other dopamine agonists may augment effects of these drugs and the effects of chasteberry itself. Conversely, if dopaminergic blockers (e.g., haloperidol) are taken concomitantly with chasteberry, the effect of the latter could be diminished. Concomitant use is not recommended.

CALCIUM—CORTICOSTEROIDS

Rating 2

RELATED DRUGS

Betamethasone

Corticotropin

Cortisone

Cosyntropin

Dexamethasone

Fludrocortisone

Hydrocortisone

Methylprednisolone

Prednisolone

Prednisone

Triamcinolone

OTHER POTENTIALLY IMPLICATED SUPPLEMENTS

Vitamin D

Interaction Summary

Corticosteroid use is associated with the accelerated development of osteoporosis. The drugs cause these effects by decreasing intestinal absorption of calcium as well as through other mechanisms. Some evidence suggests that supplementation with calcium and vitamin D may help prevent the loss of bone density associated with long-term corticosteroid therapy. However, hypercalciuria and hypercalcemia are concerns with vitamin D treatment.

Rating Scale:

(1) Significant interaction

(2) Possibly significant interaction

(3) Interaction of relatively little significance

(4) Reported interaction that does not, in fact, exist or is insignificant

Discussion

A serious side effect of long-term corticosteroid therapy (even at low dosage or by inhalation) is reduced bone density and the accelerated development of osteoporosis. Many mechanisms appear to be involved, including impaired intestinal absorption of calcium[1] and the occurrence of secondary hyperparathyroidism.[2]

Evidence suggests that calcium and vitamin D may attenuate or even reverse this loss. For example, a randomized, double-blind, placebo-controlled trial found that supplementation with calcium and vitamin D_3 prevented the loss of bone mineral density in the lumbar spine and femoral trochanter in patients taking low-dose prednisone.[1] The 2-year study involved 96 rheumatoid arthritis patients, 65 of whom were receiving low-dose corticosteroid therapy (average dose 5.6 mg/day). Patient groups were given calcium carbonate (1000 mg/day) and vitamin D_3 (500 IU/day) together or placebo. Prednisone-treated patients taking placebo *lost* bone mineral density in the lumbar spine and femoral trochanter at a yearly rate of 2% and 0.9%, respectively, whereas prednisone-treated patients taking the calcium and vitamin D_3 combination *gained* bone mineral density in those areas at a yearly rate of 0.72% and 0.85%, respectively.

A recent meta-analysis of controlled trials involving a total of 274 individuals concluded that calcium and vitamin D supplementation appear to be beneficial for corticosteroid-treated individuals.[3] Included were five randomized trials comparing calcium and vitamin D to calcium alone or placebo in patients taking systemic corticosteroids. The analysis was performed 2 years after starting calcium and vitamin D. There was a significant weighted mean difference (WMD) between treatment and control groups in lumbar (WMD 2.6; 95% CI 0.7, 4.5) and radial bone mineral density (WMD 2.5; 95% CI 0.6, 4.4). The other outcome measures (femoral neck bone mass, fracture incidence, biochemical markers of bone resorption) were not significantly different. Although the research record is not yet conclusive, the reviewers concluded that, because of the low toxicity and cost of supplementation, all patients being started on corticosteroids should receive prophylactic therapy with calcium and vitamin D.

Management Suggestions

Although evidence suggests that various vitamin D and calcium combinations may play a role in preventing corticosteroid-induced osteoporosis, vitamin D may increase the risks of hypercalciuria and hypercalcemia.[2] For this reason, corticosteroid-treated patients receiving vitamin D treatment should be closely monitored. The risk of hypercalcemia appears to be much lower with calcifediol (25-hydroxyvitamin D_3) than with calcitriol (1,25 dihydroxyvitamin D_3), the most active form of vitamin D.[4]

CALCIUM—DIGOXIN

Rating 3

RELATED DRUGS
Deslanoside   Digitoxin
Digitalis

Interaction Summary

Weak evidence suggests that digoxin may increase calcium excretion, potentially leading to depletion. The clinical significance of this finding is not known.

Discussion

Digoxin infused into a renal artery in dogs increased the urinary excretion of calcium by interfering with its reabsorption in the renal tubule.[1] The aim of this study was to clarify the renal tubular transport of calcium, magnesium, and inorganic phosphate in relation to sodium. The clinical significance of this finding was not evaluated.

Management Suggestions

Whether calcium supplementation might be helpful in patients taking digoxin is not known. On general principles, however, it would be advisable to recommend that patients obtain adequate amounts of calcium through diet or supplements.

Rating Scale:
(1) Significant interaction
(2) Possibly significant interaction

(3) Interaction of relatively little significance
(4) Reported interaction that does not, in fact, exist or is insignificant

CALCIUM—PHENYTOIN

RELATED DRUGS

Carbamazepine   Primidone
Phenobarbital

Interaction Summary

Carbamazepine and other anticonvulsant drugs may impair calcium absorption and thereby interfere with bone formation and maintenance.

Discussion

Long-term therapy with phenytoin and other anticonvulsants is associated with impaired bone formation and maintenance. The mechanism is thought to be interference with the metabolism of calcium, as well as vitamin D and vitamin K, all of which are important for proper bone status. Most studies have involved combination therapy, so it is difficult to isolate the effects of a single anticonvulsant.

Calcium absorption was compared in 12 patients on anticonvulsant therapy (all taking phenytoin and some also taking phenobarbital, primidone, and carbamazepine) and 12 controls receiving no anticonvulsants.[1] Fractional calcium absorption was

---

Rating Scale:
(1) Significant interaction
(2) Possibly significant
    interaction

(3) Interaction of relatively little
    significance
(4) Reported interaction that
    does not, in fact, exist or is
    insignificant

27% lower in the treated patients. Although phenytoin is known to impair vitamin D activity, serum levels of 25-OHD (the major circulating vitamin D metabolite) were normal, indicating that the interference of anticonvulsants with calcium absorption may be independent of an effect on vitamin D.

Weinstein et al.[2] studied 109 ambulatory adult epileptic patients receiving chronic anticonvulsant therapy (anticonvulsants included carbamazepine as well as others) and found that 48% of the patients had serum ionized calcium values below normal compared to a control group. The additional finding of normal levels of vitamin D again suggests that hypocalcemia can occur independently of anticonvulsant-induced effects on vitamin D metabolism.

Increased circulating parathyroid hormone levels were also found, indicating that the anticonvulsant-induced hypocalcemia was accompanied by secondary hyperparathyroidism, a likely compensatory mechanism; indeed, bone biopsies suggested high-turnover osteoporosis, a finding characteristic of hyperparathyroidism. The failure of this compensatory mechanism to correct the hypocalcemia suggests that anticonvulsant drugs might directly interfere with the action of parathyroid hormone.

Because hypocalcemia itself can in some cases precipitate seizures, anticonvulsant-induced hypocalcemia might result in some loss of seizure control as an additional potential consequence.

Management Suggestions

Consider calcium supplementation in patients taking anticonvulsant drugs. Note, however, that calcium carbonate might interfere with the absorption of phenytoin and perhaps other anticonvulsants.[3,4] For this reason, administer calcium supplements and anticonvulsant drugs several hours apart if possible, and monitor anticonvulsant serum levels and seizure activity.

CALCIUM—
THIAZIDE DIURETICS

Rating 1

RELATED DRUGS

Bendroflumethiazide

Benzthiazide

Chlorothiazide

Chlorthalidone

Hydrochlorothiazide

Hydroflumethiazide

Indapamide

Methylothiazide

Metolazone

Polythiazide

Quinethazone

Trichlormethiazide

Interaction Summary

Thiazide diuretics decrease urinary calcium excretion. When combined with supplemental calcium (and possibly vitamin D), this may present a risk of hypercalcemia.

Discussion

Thiazides increase calcium retention by reducing its urinary excretion, apparently through their effect on renal tubular reabsorption.[1,2] Secondary alterations in calcium intestinal absorption, parathyroid hormone secretion, and vitamin D metabolism may occur in response.

Rating Scale:

(1) Significant interaction

(2) Possibly significant interaction

(3) Interaction of relatively little significance

(4) Reported interaction that does not, in fact, exist or is insignificant

In most cases, any elevation in serum calcium is transient. However, patients taking thiazide diuretics may be at risk of significant hypercalcemia if they take calcium-containing antacids or calcium supplements. A case report described symptomatic and reversible hypercalcemia in an elderly patient taking thiazides and a calcium-containing antacid.[3] The 87-year-old woman being treated with Moduretic (HCTZ, 50 mg, and amiloride, 5 mg) was found to have been taking 6 to 8 tablets daily of an antacid formulation (calcium carbonate 680 mg and magnesium carbonate 80 mg) for many years. Clinically, she was dehydrated and constipated, and blood tests revealed hypercalcemic alkalosis, which was reversed when all medications were discontinued.

In another case a 47-year-old man was hospitalized and found to have elevated serum calcium (6.8 mEq/L) and serum creatinine (7.2 mg/dL) levels as well as metabolic alkalosis, leading to a tentative diagnosis of milk-alkali syndrome.[4] In addition to chlorothiazide, he had been taking 15 to 20 calcium carbonate tablets (500 mg each) daily for the past 2 years for heartburn. The patient's condition improved after both agents were discontinued, and he was discharged 5 days after admission.

Management Suggestions

When patients taking thiazide diuretics also use calcium supplements, monitor serum calcium and advise patients to watch for signs of hypercalcemia, such as anorexia, polydipsia, polyuria, constipation, and muscle hypotonia. This is especially important in patients also taking vitamin D and those with hyperparathyroidism.

CARBAMAZEPINE— GRAPEFRUIT JUICE

RELATED DRUGS (RATING)

Astemizole (1)

Azole antifungal agents (2)

Benzodiazepines (3)

Buspirone (2)

Calcium channel blockers (1)

Clomipramine (2)

Cyclosporine (2)

Estrogen (2)

Saquinavir mesylate (1)

Statins (1)

OTHER POTENTIALLY IMPLICATED HERBS AND SUPPLEMENTS

Cat's claw

Citrus bioflavonoids

Echinacea

Goldenseal

Licorice

St. John's wort

Wild cherry

Interaction Summary

Grapefruit juice, as a CYP enzyme–inhibitor, slows the metabolism of numerous drugs, causing a risk of excessive plasma drug levels and attendant adverse reactions. This effect may persist for 3 days or longer following the last glass of juice.

Rating Scale:

(1) Significant interaction

(2) Possibly significant interaction

(3) Interaction of relatively little significance

(4) Reported interaction that does not, in fact, exist or is insignificant

Discussion

Grapefruit juice appears to inhibit CYP3A4 enzymes, an effect that may be most important for drugs with high first-pass metabolism.[1] This inhibition can slow the normal metabolism of drugs that are substrates of this CYP enzyme system, including the anticonvulsant carbamazepine, allowing them to accumulate to potentially excessive plasma levels.[2] Constituents of grapefruit juice that may be implicated include naringenin, other flavonoids, and psoralen derivatives.[1,3]

A recent study indicates that grapefruit juice's enzyme-inhibiting effects may persist for 3 days or longer following the last glass of juice.[4] Eight healthy subjects underwent six trials, each one separated by at least a week. The first two trials consisted of a control group taking the calcium channel blocker nisoldipine, 10 mg, with water and a treatment group taking nisoldipine, 5 mg, concurrently with grapefruit juice, 200 ml. In the remaining four trials, participants drank grapefruit juice 3 times daily for 7 days, then took nisoldipine, 5 mg, at varying intervals after the last glass of juice: 12 hours, 38 hours, 72 hours, and 96 hours. Nisoldipine pharmacokinetics showed significant alterations; plasma concentration of the drug was significantly elevated in all treatment groups through the 72-hour trial, while C_{max} was significantly elevated in the concurrently treated group and in the 14-hour–treated group. In contrast, t_{max} and $t_{1/2}$ showed no significant alterations. Although the effects persisted for 72 hours, they declined as time passed and were much greater in the group ingesting drug and juice concurrently. Notably, the study used healthy volunteers, and this interaction might be expected to have greater impact in individuals taking interacting drugs for disease states.

Similar effects have been seen in vitro with numerous other herbs and plant extracts.[5]

Note on Related Drugs

Although the azole antifungal agent itraconazole is a CYP3A4 enzyme substrate, the predominant effect of its interaction appears to be *decreased* plasma drug levels caused by the inter-ference of grapefruit juice with its absorption.[2] Whether this might apply to other drugs in this family is uncertain; fluconazole, which appears not to undergo significant first-pass metabolism, may be less prone to the CYP3A4 interaction. Grapefruit juice would not be expected to affect the statin drugs fluvastatin or pravastatin because they are not metabolized by the same enzyme system. Cisapride, a discontinued drug that interacts with grapefruit juice, is not listed, but possibly some patients may still be taking it.

Management Suggestions

These findings suggest that the enzyme-inhibiting effects of regular ingestion of grapefruit juice can persist for at least 3 days and that one glass of juice is sufficient to cause an interaction. Therefore the safest approach for patients taking potentially interacting medications is to avoid grapefruit juice altogether.

CARBAMAZEPINE—
NICOTINAMIDE (NIACINAMIDE)

Rating 3

OTHER POTENTIALLY IMPLICATED SUPPLEMENTS
Niacin

Interaction Summary

Nicotinamide (niacinamide) may increase serum carbamazepine levels.

Discussion

Nicotinamide is a supplemental form of niacin that does not possess the flushing side effect or the lipid-lowering benefit of niacin. Plasma carbamazepine levels increased in two children with epilepsy after the addition of nicotinamide.[1] Clouding the issue somewhat is that these two patients were on several anti-seizure drugs concurrently. Nicotinamide may inhibit CYP450 enzymes that metabolize carbamazepine (CBZ), leading to higher drug levels. It has been proposed that this effect might be used deliberately to reduce the large fluctuations in serum CBZ levels associated with intermittent toxicity. However, the combination treatment also could lead to CBZ toxicity.

Rating Scale:
(1) Significant interaction
(2) Possibly significant interaction

(3) Interaction of relatively little significance
(4) Reported interaction that does not, in fact, exist or is insignificant

Management Suggestions

In individuals taking nicotinamide and carbamazepine, monitor serum carbamazepine concentrations and watch for signs of toxicity. Adjust the carbamazepine dose as needed.

CARNITINE—VALPROIC ACID

Rating 2

RELATED DRUGS

Barbiturates

Carbamazepine

Divalproex sodium

Phenobarbital

Phenytoin

Primidone

Valproate sodium

Interaction Summary

Long-term therapy with valproic acid, and possibly other anti-convulsant agents, may be associated with depressed carnitine levels. In most cases, the clinical significance of this effect is unclear.

Discussion

Carnitine is excreted intact by the kidneys as free carnitine or acylcarnitine, with the proximal renal tubule reabsorbing more than 90% of filtered carnitine at normal physiologic concentrations.[1] There is some evidence that valproic acid depresses the renal reabsorption of both free carnitine and acylcarnitine, although other anticonvulsants depress the renal reabsorption of acylcarnitine only.[2,3] Other mechanisms may also be involved.

Rating Scale:

(1) Significant interaction

(2) Possibly significant interaction

(3) Interaction of relatively little significance

(4) Reported interaction that does not, in fact, exist or is insignificant

In addition, many clinical studies link decreased carnitine levels to anticonvulsant therapy. The majority of these studies are in children and most involve valproic acid.[1]

However, most of the reports thus far have significant limitations.[4] Generally, carnitine levels were not measured before initiation of drug therapy, so these levels could have already been low in some patients. For this reason, it is uncertain whether the disease, the treatment, a combination of both, or other factors exert this effect on carnitine levels.

One study did measure blood carnitine levels before and after anticonvulsant therapy in 37 children.[5] Total carnitine levels in the valproic acid group declined from 45.3 μM before treatment to 34.9 μM after treatment. In the carbamazepine group, carnitine levels decreased from 45.7 μM to 43.4 μM, and in the phenobarbital group, from 44.9 μM to 42.1 μM. Only the children taking valproic acid showed a significant decrease ($P < 0.001$) in their baseline carnitine levels.

In a study involving 183 adult outpatients and 49 control subjects, a deficiency of free carnitine (defined as more than 2 standard deviations below the mean) was found in 77% of those taking valproic acid.[6] This deficiency was found in 27% of subjects taking phenytoin plus phenobarbital, 23% of those taking carbamazepine, and 16% of those taking phenytoin.

The evidence is not entirely consistent, however. Another study, in 471 children of various ages on anticonvulsant therapy compared to 32 healthy children aged 1 to 16 years serving as controls, found more significantly reduced carnitine levels with phenobarbital monotherapy than with valproic acid monotherapy.[7] The following percentages of patients on monotherapy were found to be deficient in total and free carnitine: phenobarbital (36% total; 21% free), valproic acid (23% total; 9% free), phenytoin (12% total; 8% free), carbamazepine (8% total; 1% free). For those on polytherapy, the percentages were valproic acid/carbamazepine (44% total; 22% free), phenobarbital/phenytoin (37% total; 16% free), phenobarbital/carbamazepine (18% total; 6% free).

Carnitine supplementation does appear to normalize low carnitine levels associated with anticonvulsant therapy. A case-control study evaluated 41 epileptic children—14 on valproic acid monotherapy and 27 on valproic acid polytherapy—along with 41 age- and sex-matched healthy control participants.[8] Mean total and free carnitine levels were significantly lower in both treatment groups compared to controls. Although there were no statistically significant differences in carnitine concentrations between the two treatment groups, those on valproic acid polytherapy had slightly lower carnitine levels than those on valproic acid monotherapy; carnitine deficiency was related to duration of valproic acid treatment, but not to blood levels of valproic acid. Supplementation with L-carnitine in 11 patients with low levels of carnitine significantly increased serum free and total carnitine concentrations and normalized them.

Carnitine depletion has been hypothesized to contribute to valproic acid hepatotoxicity.[9] Valproic acid–induced carnitine depletion may help explain the drug's known interference with fatty acid oxidation. In a study measuring energy metabolism in children receiving long-term treatment with valproic acid, researchers compared 10 randomly selected subjects to age- and sex-matched controls.[10] Eight of the treated subjects showed an altered energy consumption pattern, including a significant reduction in the amount of fats oxidized and a shift to increased utilization of carbohydrates. Carnitine supplementation for a month (50 mg/kg/day as an oral solution, divided equally into 2 or 3 doses) appeared to reverse this pattern. Younger children (1 to 10 years) treated with valproic acid may experience a more pronounced decrease in carnitine concentrations than older children (10 to 18 years).[1]

However, no symptomatic benefits were seen with carnitine supplementation in a double-blind, placebo-controlled crossover study. Freeman et al.[4] examined the effects of carnitine supplementation (100 mg/kg daily) in 37 children (ages 3 to 17 years) with epilepsy who were taking valproic acid or carbamazepine.

The study was designed to assess patients' "well-being" as perceived by their parents. No significant improvement was noted.

Management Suggestions

L-Carnitine supplementation may be advisable in certain cases, such as infants and young children receiving valproic acid, especially those younger than 2 years who are receiving anticonvulsant polytherapy. One general dosing recommendation is to administer oral carnitine in 3 or 4 divided doses for a total daily dose of 100 mg/kg or 2 g, whichever is less.[1]

CHROMIUM—
CALCIUM CARBONATE

Rating 3

Interaction Summary

Antacids containing calcium carbonate may reduce the absorption of chromium when the two are taken together.

Discussion

Measuring chromium status in humans is difficult, but a study in rats using an isotope of chromium made possible a sensitive evaluation of a potential calcium-chromium interaction.[1] The findings suggest that calcium carbonate may reduce the absorption and tissue retention of chromium from orally ingested chromium chloride. The mechanism of this interaction is unclear but may involve pH levels, formation of insoluble complexes, or both.

Management Suggestions

Since marginal chromium status may be common in humans,[2] this interaction could be important. To minimize potential problems, administer calcium-containing antacids or calcium supplements (especially calcium carbonate) 2 to 3 hours apart from chromium supplements and meals.

Rating Scale:
(1) Significant interaction
(2) Possibly significant interaction

(3) Interaction of relatively little significance
(4) Reported interaction that does not, in fact, exist or is insignificant

CIPROFLOXACIN—FENNEL

Rating 2

RELATED DRUGS

Enoxacin	Ofloxacin
Grepafloxacin	Sparfloxacin
Lomefloxacin	Trovalfloxacin
Norfloxacin	

Interaction Summary

The herb fennel appears to alter ciprofloxacin bioavailability and pharmacokinetics, potentially impairing its effectiveness. Similar effects may be expected with other fluoroquinolones.

Discussion

In a placebo-controlled study in rats, potential interactions between ciprofloxacin and oral doses of the herb fennel were evaluated.[1] Fennel was found to reduce the maximum plasma concentration, AUC, and urinary excretion of ciprofloxacin by 83%, 48%, and 43%, respectively. Bioavailability was reduced by about 50%, and volume of distribution and terminal elimination half-life were significantly increased.

The mechanism of this interaction is not clear, although it may involve metal ions found in fennel.

Rating Scale:
(1) Significant interaction
(2) Possibly significant interaction

(3) Interaction of relatively little significance
(4) Reported interaction that does not, in fact, exist or is insignificant

Management Suggestions

Allowing 2 hours between ciprofloxacin and fennel intake should reduce the potential for interactions, but may not eliminate it. For this reason, it may be advisable to avoid fennel supplementation during treatment with ciprofloxacin or other fluoroquinolones.

CLOMIPRAMINE—SAMe

RELATED DRUGS

Amitriptyline

Amoxapine

Citalopram

Desipramine

Doxepin

Fluoxetine

Fluvoxamine

Imipramine

Isocarboxazid

Naratriptan

Nefazodone

Nortriptyline

Paroxetine

Phenelzine

Protroptyline

Rizatriptan

Sertraline

Sumatriptain

Tramadol

Tranylcypromine

Trimipramine

Venlafaxine

Zolmitriptan

OTHER POTENTIALLY IMPLICATED SUPPLEMENTS

5-HTP

Interaction Summary

Based on one case report involving agents that increase serotonin activity, combining S-adenosylmethionine (SAMe) with other drugs that elevate serotonin could cause serotonin

Rating Scale:
(1) Significant interaction
(2) Possibly significant interaction

(3) Interaction of relatively little significance
(4) Reported interaction that does not, in fact, exist or is insignificant

syndrome. These include MAO inhibitors, SSRIs, tricyclics, and antimigraine drugs.

Discussion

The case report involved a possible toxic interaction between the tricyclic antidepressant clomipramine and SAMe that appeared to involve increased CNS serotonin activity.[1] A 71-year-old woman with a history of major affective disorder had received SAMe 100 mg/day IM and clomipramine 25 mg/day for 10 days. At that time the clomipramine dose was increased to 75 mg/day. She became progressively anxious, agitated, and confused, and 2 to 3 days later was admitted to the hospital verbally unresponsive and stuporous along with other symptoms. The syndrome resolved over a few days with hydration and supportive care, and the patient completely recovered.

Serotonin syndrome was diagnosed based on laboratory tests and other information. The condition was believed to be due to the synergistic action of SAMe and clomipramine in increasing CNS serotonin activity. Clomipramine increases CNS serotonin activity more than any other tricyclic antidepressant. Although SAMe is not known to affect serotonin, it is believed to have antidepressant activity, and its mechanism of action for that effect is not known.

Most antidepressant drugs have some serotonergic effects. In addition, the nonnarcotic analgesic tramadol (Ultram) affects serotonin and has been associated with serotonin syndrome.[2,3]

The supplement 5-HTP is a serotonin precursor, and as such could also potentially contribute to serotonin syndrome.

Management Suggestions

It may be advisable to avoid combining the supplements SAMe or 5-HTP with drugs that elevate serotonin levels.

CLONIDINE—YOHIMBE (SOURCE OF YOHIMBINE)

Rating 2

RELATED DRUGS

ACE inhibitors	Calcium channel blockers
Alpha-adrenergic–blocking agents	CNS stimulants
	MAO inhibitors
Antihypertensives	Phenothiazines
Beta-blockers	Tricyclics

Interaction Summary

Yohimbine, the primary active ingredient in the herb yohimbe, may increase blood pressure, offsetting the antihypertensive effects of established antihypertensives (e.g., beta-blockers and calcium channel blockers). Additionally, a potential interaction exists with clonidine that may result in increased blood pressure. Yohimbine may also interact with tricyclic antidepressants, MAO inhibitors, CNS stimulants, phenothiazines, and alpha-adrenergic–blocking agents, acting to either increase or decrease blood pressure.

Rating Scale:
(1) Significant interaction
(2) Possibly significant interaction
(3) Interaction of relatively little significance
(4) Reported interaction that does not, in fact, exist or is insignificant

Discussion

Yohimbine has been advocated to decrease blood pressure.[1] However, yohimbine has been shown to in fact increase blood pressure when taken in doses exceeding 5 mg.[1] Yohimbine apparently increases norepinephrine release into the bloodstream by direct stimulation of sympathetic outflow from the brain as well as blockade of inhibitory alpha$_2$-adrenergic receptors on sympathetic nerve endings, enhancing the amount of norepinephrine release for a given amount of sympathetic traffic.[2]

Following oral doses of 20 or 40 mg of yohimbine to normal young men, yohimbine caused a dose-dependent increase in plasma epinephrine, presumably resulting from increased epinephrine release from the adrenals.[3] Systolic and diastolic blood pressures increased 10 ± 2 (range: 4 to 26) and 5 ± 1 (range: 2 to 17) mm Hg, respectively, in a study of 25 white adult patients with uncomplicated essential hypertension who were administered yohimbine at 21.6 mg.[4] This has been confirmed in a study of 59 subjects in which yohimbine caused a mean increase in systolic blood pressure of 7 ± 14 mm Hg 120 minutes after administration.[5] In a yohimbine bolus challenge test, the mean arterial pressure increased $13\% \pm 2\%$ in normotensive patients and $17\% \pm 2\%$ in hypertensive patients.[2]

It would thus appear that hypertensive patients are more prone to the hypertensive effects of yohimbine. This has been confirmed elsewhere in a study of 25 healthy volunteers and 29 gender- and age-matched untreated hypertensive patients; no significant effect was noted in normotensive patients, but a significant ($P < 0.05$) increase in diastolic pressure was noted at the tenth minute of upright posture.[6]

Hence, although not yet observed in clinical practice, it is possible that yohimbine diminishes the blood-pressure–lowering effect of antihypertensive agents. More specifically, the effects of clonidine may be directly blocked by yohimbine. Yohimbine has been found to block inhibitory alpha$_2$-adrenergic receptors on vascular smooth muscles, causing reflexive increases in sympathetic outflow.[2] This mechanism of action directly interferes with clonidine, which is a central alpha$_2$-adrenergic agonist that inhibits sympathetic outflow from the central nervous system and decreases peripheral resistance, heart rate, and blood pressure.[7]

Neither in vitro studies nor clinical observational studies have been conducted to examine this interaction, but its potential has been noted.[8,9] This interaction may be more profound if yohimbine is taken with monoamine oxidase inhibitors because this furthers the effects of endogenous sympathomimetic amines, increasing blood pressure. However, again, documentation is lacking.

Although benzodiazepines are not antihypertensive agents, alprazolam (but not diazepam) has been shown to decrease systolic and diastolic blood pressure; this effect was antagonized by yohimbine administration in healthy subjects.[10,11] Furthermore, yohimbine's blood pressure effect has been used to therapeutic advantage to offset orthostasis associated with clomipramine and despiramine.[12-14]

Management Suggestions

Prudence dictates close monitoring of blood pressure if yohimbe herb is added to an antihypertensive regimen.

COENZYME Q_{10}— ACETOHEXAMIDE

Rating 3

RELATED DRUGS

Chlorpropamide Phenformin
Glipizide   Tolazamide
Glyburide   Tolbutamide

Interaction Summary

Some oral hypoglycemic drugs appear to inhibit the activity of coenzyme Q_{10} (CoQ_{10}) and may worsen an existing deficiency of CoQ_{10} in patients with diabetes. CoQ_{10} supplementation may reduce glucose levels.

Discussion

The mean percent deficiency of CoQ_{10} was significantly greater (20% $\pm$ 0.7%) in 120 patients with diabetes than in healthy controls (16% $\pm$ 1.0%), based on measuring the activity of the CoQ_{10} enzyme succinate dehydrogenase–CoQ_{10} reductase in leukocytes from blood samples.[1] Additionally, in order of decreasing effect, the hypoglycemic drugs acetohexamide, glyburide, phenformin, and tolazamide inhibited the CoQ_{10} enzyme NADH-oxidase in test tube preparations. The hypoglycemic drugs tolbutamide, glipizide, and chlorpropamide had no inhibitory effect on NADH-oxidase or the CoQ_{10} enzyme succinoxidase.

Rating Scale:

(1) Significant interaction
(2) Possibly significant interaction

(3) Interaction of relatively little significance
(4) Reported interaction that does not, in fact, exist or is insignificant

Of the drugs phenformin, tolazamide, glipizide, and tolbutamide, it was determined that the incidence of CoQ_{10} deficiency was significantly higher in patients taking phenformin and tolazamide than in controls, although some of these patients also were taking one other drug. Patients taking the stronger CoQ_{10} enzyme inhibitors acetohexamide and glyburide might also be expected to show a significant incidence of CoQ_{10} deficiency compared to controls.

A CoQ_{10} deficiency in some of these patients with diabetes cannot be solely attributed to inhibitory effects of the drugs, however, because a group of 37 diabetic patients whose disease was controlled by diet alone showed a mean percent deficiency of $20.2\% \pm 1.3\%$, which was significantly greater than controls. However, it seems reasonable to think that a preexisting CoQ_{10} deficiency would be enhanced by CoQ_{10}-inhibitory antidiabetic drugs. A deficiency of CoQ_{10} in the pancreas could impair bioenergetics, ATP generation, and insulin biosynthesis.

A randomized, double-blind trial involving patients with hypertension and coronary artery disease found that supplementation with 60 mg of CoQ_{10} twice daily was associated with a significant decline in fasting and 2-hour plasma insulin and glucose levels compared to controls.[2] For this reason, it may be necessary to reduce oral hypoglycemic doses in patients who start CoQ_{10} supplementation.

Management Suggestions

Patients taking certain oral hypoglycemics may benefit from supplementation. A typical supplemental dose of CoQ_{10} is 30 to 100 mg daily.

Because CoQ_{10} supplementation may reduce glucose levels, it may be necessary to reduce the oral hypoglycemic dose if CoQ_{10} is added. Monitor blood glucose levels carefully and adjust the dose of the oral hypoglycemic drug as needed in patients taking this combination. Advise patients to report signs of hypoglycemia, including acute fatigue, restlessness, malaise, marked irritability, and weakness.

COENZYME Q$_{10}$—CHLORPROMAZINE

Rating 3

RELATED DRUGS

Phenothiazines
  Acetophenazine
  Fluphenazine
  Mesoridazine
  Methotrimeprazine
  Perphenazine
  Prochlorperazine
  Promazine
  Promethazine
  Propiomazine
  Thiethylperazine
  Thioridazine

Trifluoperazine
Triflupromazine
Tricyclic antidepressants
  Amitriptyline
  Amoxapine
  Clomipramine
  Desipramine
  Doxepin
  Imipramine
  Nortriptyline
  Protriptyline
  Trimipramine

Interaction Summary

Phenothiazines and tricyclic antidepressants have been reported to inhibit enzymes containing coenzyme Q$_{10}$ (CoQ$_{10}$).

Rating Scale:
(1) Significant interaction
(2) Possibly significant interaction

(3) Interaction of relatively little significance
(4) Reported interaction that does not, in fact, exist or is insignificant

Discussion

The vitamin-like substance CoQ$_{10}$ (ubiquinone) is present naturally in cardiac muscle and other tissues and appears to play a fundamental role in producing the mitochondrial cell energy needed for normal heart function.[1] Folkers[2] noted that Kishi et al.[3] summarized extensive data on the inhibition of myocardial respiration by psychotherapeutic drugs and its prevention by CoQ$_{10}$. Phenothiazines and tricyclic antidepressants were found to inhibit the CoQ$_{10}$ enzymes NADH-oxidase and succinoxidase in test tube studies.[3]

Management Suggestions

Based on these inhibitory effects, it has been suggested that CoQ$_{10}$ supplementation might help prevent the myocardial-depressant effects associated with phenothiazines and the cardiac-related adverse effects associated with tricyclic antidepressants. However, this has not been proved. A typical supplemental dose of CoQ$_{10}$ is 30 to 100 mg daily.

COENZYME Q_{10}—LOVASTATIN

Rating 2

RELATED DRUGS

Atorvastatin   Pravastatin

Cerivastatin   Simvastatin

Fluvastatin

Interaction Summary

Statin drugs lower coenzyme Q_{10} (CoQ_{10}) levels along with cholesterol. Inadequate CoQ_{10} levels may adversely affect cardiac function and other fundamental energy processes in the body.

Discussion

The vitamin-like substance CoQ_{10} (ubiquinone) is an endogenous antioxidant and an essential component of the electron-transfer system in mitochondrial membranes.[1,2] It is present in cardiac muscle and other tissues and appears to play a fundamental role in producing the mitochondrial cell energy needed for normal heart function.[3] Statin drugs work by inhibiting HMG-CoA reductase, an enzyme necessary for the synthesis of cholesterol and CoQ_{10}. For this reason, statins tend to lower serum levels of CoQ_{10} along with cholesterol. It has been reported that statins do not completely inhibit HMG-CoA reductase and that necessary amounts of CoQ_{10} may still be

---

Rating Scale:

(1) Significant interaction

(2) Possibly significant interaction

(3) Interaction of relatively little significance

(4) Reported interaction that does not, in fact, exist or is insignificant

synthesized. However, several studies suggest that the extent of statin-induced CoQ$_{10}$ loss may be clinically important.

A randomized, double-blind, placebo-controlled trial involving 45 hypercholesterolemic patients taking lovastatin or pravastatin over an 18-week period found a significant dose-related decline of total serum CoQ$_{10}$ levels associated with both drugs.[2] Serum levels of CoQ$_{10}$ were measured parallel to cholesterol levels at baseline, with placebo and diet, and during active treatment. Compared to baseline, lovastatin 20 to 80 mg/day produced a 29% decrease in serum CoQ$_{10}$, while pravastatin 10 to 40 mg/day produced a 19.7% decrease.

Similarly, a 3-month, double-blind, placebo-controlled study found that treatment with simvastatin or pravastatin 20 mg/day lowered CoQ$_{10}$ plasma levels in 30 hypercholesterolemic patients as well as 10 normal volunteers.[1] After 12 weeks of treatment, initial CoQ$_{10}$ levels were lowered by 54% with simvastatin and 50% with pravastatin. This could be clinically important, especially in patients with higher metabolic CoQ$_{10}$ requirements.

Furthermore, statin-induced lowering of CoQ$_{10}$ tissue levels appears to depress cardiac function to variable degrees.[4] Five hospitalized patients (43 to 72 years old) with cardiomyopathy who were treated with lovastatin showed decreased CoQ$_{10}$ blood levels and deterioration of cardiac function, including a worsening of the ejection fraction. Subsequent oral supplementation with CoQ$_{10}$ (100 to 200 mg/day) led to increased CoQ$_{10}$ blood levels and a reversal of the cardiac deterioration.

Another study found that supplemental CoQ$_{10}$ could prevent plasma and platelet CoQ$_{10}$ reduction without affecting the therapeutic effect of simvastatin.[5] In this 3-month study involving 30 patients with primary hypercholesterolemia (IIa phenotype), one group took 20 mg of simvastain and one group took 20 mg of simvastain plus 100 mg of CoQ$_{10}$. The statin-only group showed a 26% decrease in plasma CoQ$_{10}$ levels (from 1.08

mg/dl to 0.8 mg/dl). In contrast, the CoQ_{10}-supplemented group showed a significant 23.3% increase in plasma CoQ_{10} (from 1.2 mg/dl to 1.48 mg/dl). Cholesterol-lowering effects were similar in both groups. Platelet CoQ_{10} also decreased in the statin-only group by 13.5% (from 104 to 90 ng/mg) and increased in the CoQ_{10}-supplemented group by 52.6% (from 95 to 145 ng/mg).

Management Suggestions

Consider CoQ_{10} supplementation in patients taking statin drugs, especially those with compromised cardiac function.

COENZYME Q$_{10}$—PROPRANOLOL

Rating 2

RELATED DRUGS

Beta-blockers
  Acebutolol
  Atenolol
  Betaxolol
  Bisoprolol
  Carteolol
  Esmolol
  Metoprolol
  Nadolol
  Penbutolol
  Pindolol
  Propranolol
  Sotalol
  Timolol

Other antihypertensive drugs
  Bendroflumethiazide
  Benzthiazide
  Chlorothiazide
  Chlorthalidone
  Clonidine
  Hydralazine
  Hydrochlorothiazide
  Hydroflumethiazide
  Indapamide
  Methyclothiazide
  Methyldopa
  Metolazone
  Polythiazide
  Quinethazone
  Trichlormethiazide

Interaction Summary

Based on in vitro studies, various antihypertensive drugs, particularly the beta-blocker propranolol, appear to inhibit enzymes containing CoQ$_{10}$ in heart muscle tissue. The depressed

Rating Scale:
(1) Significant interaction
(2) Possibly significant interaction
(3) Interaction of relatively little significance
(4) Reported interaction that does not, in fact, exist or is insignificant

myocardial function (e.g., diminish myocardial contractility and cardiac output) observed with beta-blocker drugs may cause significant fatigue, especially in elderly patients, and could be related to drug-induced inhibition of CoQ_{10} enzymes in the myocardium. This effect could be especially significant in patients with a preexisting CoQ_{10} deficiency. Of the beta-blockers, timolol showed negligible inhibition.

Discussion

The vitamin-like substance CoQ_{10} (ubiquinone) is present naturally in cardiac muscle and other tissues and appears to play a fundamental role in producing the mitochondrial cell energy needed for normal heart function.[1] Energy deficiency of heart muscle cells is believed to be one of the numerous possible causes of myocardial dysfunction and may play a significant role in the progression of heart failure. CoQ_{10} levels have been found to be significantly decreased in patients with myocardial failure (dilated and restrictive cardiomyopathy and alcoholic heart disease) compared to normal myocardium. The more severe the disease, the lower the tissue levels of CoQ_{10}. In an open study of 40 patients in severe heart failure (classes III and IV), nearly two thirds showed objective and subjective improvement when treated with 100 mg of CoQ_{10} daily. CoQ_{10} deficiencies have also been found in hypertensive patients taking antihypertensive drugs and those not taking them.[2]

Based on assays for drug-induced inhibition of enzymes containing CoQ_{10} in mitochondrial preparations from beef heart, various antihypertensive drugs were found to have an inhibiting effect.[2] Of the beta-blockers, propranolol substantially inhibited the CoQ_{10} enzyme NADH-oxidase, metoprolol was less inhibitory than propranolol, and timolol showed negligible inhibition, which correlates with timolol's low cardiac depressant effects. Another in vitro study of antihypertensive drugs found similar results[2]: propranolol was the greatest inhibitor of NADH-oxidase; metoprolol, which is structurally similar to propranolol, showed 25% as much inhibition. Additionally, of 268 hospitalized patients receiving propranolol, about 10% had adverse reactions related to depressed myocardial function associated with the drug, and some of the side effects occurred at a dose of 30 mg daily or less.

In an open study, three of five subjects taking propranolol complained of general malaise, while none of seven subjects taking a combination of propranolol and CoQ_{10} reported this side effect.[3] The depressed myocardial function associated with propranolol could be at least partly related to the drug's inhibition of CoQ_{10} enzymes in the myocardium.[2] Based on these findings, it is possible that a preexisting deficiency of CoQ_{10} in the myocardium of hypertensive patients could be worsened by propranolol therapy.[2]

Of the other antihypertensive drugs, the inhibitory effects of clonidine and hydralazine on NADH-oxidase were similar to that of metoprolol, which showed 25% as much inhibition as propranolol.[2] The inhibitory effect of hydrochlorothiazide was slightly less. Methyldopa very weakly inhibited the CoQ_{10} enzyme succinoxidase and had no significant effect on NADH-oxidase. Although the inhibitory action of these drugs falls well below that of propranolol, this effect may merit consideration for patients on these antihypertensives.

Management Suggestions

CoQ_{10} supplementation may help counteract side effects associated with the depressed myocardial function seen with propranolol and perhaps other beta-blockers. The benefit of CoQ_{10} supplementation in patients taking other antihypertensive drugs is unknown, although it might be helpful in patients with a preexisting CoQ_{10} deficiency. A typical supplemental dose of CoQ_{10} is 30 to 100 mg daily.

COPPER—ORAL CONTRACEPTIVES

Rating 3

Interaction Summary

Oral contraceptives (OCs) appear to increase serum copper concentrations. Third-generation OCs may elevate serum copper levels to a greater extent, possibly because of the newer progestins they contain.

Discussion

Epidemiologic studies have demonstrated an association between OC use and elevated copper levels. In one study, plasma copper concentrations were significantly higher in women than in men and were higher in women taking OCs.[1] Another study found that OC use was associated with elevated serum copper and ferritin values and lowered serum magnesium levels.[2]

Progestins in OCs are believed to be the primary determinant of elevated copper levels. An epidemiologic study of 610 women aged 18 to 44 years determined that higher serum copper concentrations in women using OCs was more strongly linked to progestin content than to estrogen.[3] The greatest increase in serum copper levels, compared to non-users of OCs, occurred in women taking OCs containing antiandrogen progestins (56% increase), followed by desogestrel (46%), norethisteron/lynestrenol (42%), and levonorgestrel (34%), after adjusting for

---

Rating Scale:

(1) Significant interaction

(2) Possibly significant interaction

(3) Interaction of relatively little significance

(4) Reported interaction that does not, in fact, exist or is insignificant

multiple covariates (e.g., age, smoking, alcohol use). Serum copper concentrations differed only marginally in relation to estrogen content. Use of OCs containing lower doses of ethylestradiol was associated with a greater increase in serum copper levels; however, this could reflect the fact that newer progestins are used in combination with low-dose ethylestradiol.

This elevation in copper concentrations might be of clinical significance. Epidemiologic studies suggest an increased mortality from cardiovascular diseases in individuals with higher serum copper levels, although a causal association has not been proved. In a nested case-control study within a prospective population study, high serum copper and low serum zinc concentrations were significantly associated with an increased mortality from all cardiovascular diseases and from coronary heart disease in particular.[4] Another epidemiologic study suggested that high copper status, reflected by elevated serum copper concentration, may be an independent risk factor for ischemic heart disease.[5]

Management Suggestions

Although epidemiologic evidence suggests that high serum copper concentration is associated with increased cardiovascular risk, it does not prove a causal association. Whether to monitor copper concentrations in patients taking OCs is therefore unclear at this time.

CORTICOSTEROIDS— CHROMIUM

Rating 2

RELATED DRUGS

Betamethasone	Methylprednisolone
Cortisone acetate	Prednisolone
Dexamethasone	Prednisone
Hydrocortisone	Triamcinolone

Interaction Summary

Chromium supplementation may help control corticosteroid-induced diabetes.

Discussion

A 1999 study demonstrates that supplementation with the trace mineral chromium may help control corticosteroid-induced diabetes.[1] Corticosteroid therapy is known to cause decreased insulin sensitivity, impaired glucose tolerance, and/or diabetes, and evidence suggests that chromium supplementation has a positive effect on these conditions.[2-5]

Ravina et al.[1] administered chromium picolinate at a dose of 200 μg 3 times daily (total 600 μg) to patients with uncontrolled corticosteroid-induced diabetes. Within 1 week, blood glucose values in 47 of the 50 patients decreased from the baseline of

---

Rating Scale:

(1) Significant interaction

(2) Possibly significant interaction

(3) Interaction of relatively little significance

(4) Reported interaction that does not, in fact, exist or is insignificant

greater than 13.9 mmol/L to less than 8.3 mmol/L despite the fact that oral antidiabetic drug or insulin dose was reduced by half prior to starting chromium. After 2 weeks, supplemental chromium intake was reduced to 200 μg daily. In three patients who discontinued chromium and medication, blood glucose levels increased but returned to acceptable levels on restoration of chromium, at the maintenance dose of 200 μg daily.

Management Suggestions

Supplemental chromium may be useful in the prevention and control of corticosteroid-induced diabetes.

CYCLOSPORINE—ECHINACEA

Rating 2

RELATED DRUGS

Azathioprine
Basiliximab
Corticosteroids
Daclizumab

Muromonab
Mycophenolate
Tacrolimus

OTHER POTENTIALLY IMPLICATED HERBS

Andrographis
Ashwagandha
Astragalus
Garlic
Ginseng *(Panax ginseng)*

Maitake
Reishi
Schisandra
Suma

Interaction Summary

The apparent immunomodulating effects of echinacea might diminish the effectiveness of cyclosporine and other immunosuppressants.

Discussion

Echinacea has been advocated as an immunostimulant for various conditions, such as the common cold and other upper respiratory infections.[1,2] Evidence suggests that it might increase

Rating Scale:

(1) Significant interaction
(2) Possibly significant interaction

(3) Interaction of relatively little significance
(4) Reported interaction that does not, in fact, exist or is insignificant

interferon-alpha, interferon-beta, tumor necrosis factor-alpha, and IgM levels.[3] In concentrations down to 1 μg/ml, echinacea strongly activated macrophages in mice as measured by specific ^{51}Cr release from p815 tumor cells (62% $\pm$ 4% versus 28% $\pm$ 3% ^{51}Cr release in the control medium).[4]

However, in five placebo-controlled, randomized studies involving 134 healthy volunteers, the actual number of white blood cells was unaffected.[5] In this same report it was noted that the phagocytic activity of polymorphonuclear neutrophil granulocytes (PNG) was enhanced (maximal stimulation 23% to 54%) in only two of five studies. Nonetheless, the potential exists for an adverse herb-drug interaction if echinacea is combined with any drug intended for immunosuppression such as cyclosporine or tacrolimus. Generally, these agents are administered to prevent organ rejection following transplantation. Interference with the efficacy of these drugs could have life-threatening consequences for these patients. Hence, stimulating the immune system with echinacea might be problematic.

Management Suggestions

Patients should be advised to avoid echinacea use immediately before, during, and after transplantation when azathioprine, basiliximab, cyclosporine, daclizumab, muromonab, mycophenolate, or tacrolimus may be used for immunosuppression.

CYCLOSPORINE—IPRIFLAVONE

Rating 2

RELATED DRUGS

Corticosteroids
Methotrexate

Other immunosuppressants

Interaction Summary

Ipriflavone might decrease leukocyte count, potentiating the action of immunosuppressant drugs.

Discussion

Ipriflavone is a semisynthetic phytoestrogen used to treat osteoporosis. In a 3-year study of 474 postmenopausal women, ipriflavone use was associated with decreased lymphocyte levels, reaching lymphopenia in 29 participants.[1] Similar effects were seen in another much smaller study.[2] The cause and clinical significance of this finding is not clear.

Management Suggestions

Ipriflavone should be used with caution in individuals taking immunosuppressant drugs.

Rating Scale:

(1) Significant interaction
(2) Possibly significant interaction

(3) Interaction of relatively little significance
(4) Reported interaction that does not, in fact, exist or is insignificant

CYCLOSPORINE—
ST. JOHN'S WORT

Rating 1

NOTE: See Table I in Guengerich for the most comprehensive list of CYP3A4 and p-glycoprotein drug substrates.[1]

RELATED DRUGS

CYP3A4 and
P-glycoprotein
Drug substrates, including
cyclosporine, digoxin,
warfarin, oral contraceptives,
theophylline, simvastatin,
lovastatin, and atorvastatin
(but not pravastatin)

Saquinavir
Indinavir

Interaction Summary

Concomitant use of St. John's wort extract causes increased metabolism, and possibly impaired absorption, of the immunosuppressive drug cyclosporine.

Discussion

Swiss investigators described two heart transplant patients in their early 60s who exhibited signs of acute transplant rejection at 11 and 20 months after transplantation.[2] Both individuals had been maintained successfully on nearly identical

Rating Scale:
(1) Significant interaction
(2) Possibly significant
    interaction

(3) Interaction of relatively little
    significance
(4) Reported interaction that
    does not, in fact, exist or is
    insignificant

immunosuppressive regimens of cyclosporine, azathioprine, and corticosteroids.

Three weeks before admission for transplant rejection, they had each started therapy with the European St. John's wort extract, LI160 (Jarsin), 300 mg 3 times daily. Medical records showed that both patients had previously maintained therapeutic plasma cyclosporine levels of 200 to 260 μg/L, but at this time were well below therapeutic levels (95 and 87 μg/L, respectively).

On discontinuation of St. John's wort, cyclosporine levels increased to above 200 μg/L in both patients, and no further episodes of rejection were observed. These authors considered the possibility that St. John's wort may have induced the activity of hepatic CYP3A4, causing decreased plasma levels of the 3A4 substrate, cyclosporine. However, the authors also hypothesized that St. John's wort–mediated induction of p-glycoprotein (hypothesized to have increased digoxin clearance by Johne et al.[3]) could also have contributed to decreased cyclosporine oral bioavailability.

In another report, 35 kidney transplant and 10 liver transplant recipients were noted to have an average 49% fall in cyclosporine levels after starting St. John's wort, and two rejection episodes occurred.[4] These reports have been confirmed by independent observations.[5]

Increasing evidence indicates that St. John's wort induces CYP3A and intestinal p-glycoprotein.[6,7] For example, one trial found that St. John's wort decreased plasma concentrations of simvastatin but not pravastatin.[8] Simvastatin is metabolized by CYP3A4 in the gut and liver, while pravastatin is primarily metabolized through non-CYP pathways.

It should be noted that there exists one high-quality but small prospective study suggesting that St. John's wort is *without* significant effect on CYP3A4 or another major cytochrome P-450, CYP2D6.[9] The discrepancy between this and other reports may be due to the variable quality of St. John's wort preparations used in each study. In addition, another report using urinary 6-beta-hydroxycortisol/cortisol ratios as a measure of CYP3A4 activity in human volunteers before and after 14 days of St. John's wort revealed large interindividual variations in CYP3A4 induction among subjects (mean 114% ± 95% change from baseline, range of –25% to 259%).[10]

Hypericin is most likely the St. John's wort component that mediates CYP1A2 induction.[11] The compound responsible for CYP3A4 induction appears to be hyperforin, one of the proposed active ingredients in the herb. Of 15 St. John's wort components tested, hyperforin was the only one shown to induce CYP3A4 in human hepatocytes.[12] This effect appears to be mediated by hyperforin binding to and activating the hepatic transcription factor PXR. In fact, hyperforin is at least 50-fold more potent in binding PXR than rifampicin, the classical CYP3A4 inducer. This report raises another issue: the known chemical instability of hyperforin may partly account for the variable CYP3A4 induction observed with different St. John's wort preparations.

Management Suggestions

As with any life-threatening condition, patients who are candidates for organ transplant are predisposed to depression. Such individuals may choose to self-medicate with St. John's wort in the false belief that because it is "natural," it is safe. The result may be inadequate treatment. Conversely, if drug levels are adjusted in an individual already taking St. John's wort, abrupt discontinuation of the herb could result in rebound toxicity. Physician vigilance is warranted. Direct questioning and counseling is advised because patients may not volunteer information regarding their use of herbs.

DIGOXIN—FOXGLOVE

Rating 1

OTHER POTENTIALLY IMPLICATED HERBS

Adonis

Dogbane

False hellebore

Lily of the valley

Milkweed

Motherwort

Oleander

Pheasant's eye

Pleurisy root

Strophanthus

Uzara root

White squill

Wild ipecac

Interaction Summary

Digoxin-type effects may be exacerbated if digoxin is used with foxglove. Although foxglove is not used as a medicinal herb today, other herbs that contain cardiac glycosides could cause similar problems.

Discussion

Several herbs listed above contain appreciable amounts of cardiac glycosides. Leaves of wild varieties of these herbs used for medicinal purposes have been found to contain 30 different glycosides in quantities ranging from 0.1% to 0.6%, although contaminants may have occurred in some cases.[1] No reports exist documenting adverse effects of concomitant use in human be-

---

Rating Scale:

(1) Significant interaction

(2) Possibly significant interaction

(3) Interaction of relatively little significance

(4) Reported interaction that does not, in fact, exist or is insignificant

ings. If encountered, however, cardiac glycoside poisoning manifests as blurred vision, strong but slowed pulse, nausea, vomiting, dizziness, frequent urination, and contracted pupils. In severe cases, fatigue, confusion, stupor, and cardiac disturbances (including arrhythmias) can occur. Because of the structural and pharmacologic similarity between digoxin and cardiac glycosides found in oleander (e.g., oleandrin, neriine, oleandroside, nerioside, and digitoxigenin), digoxin-specific Fab fragments (Digibind) can be successfully used to treat oleander toxicity.[2]

Management Suggestions

Herbs containing cardiac glycosides can augment digoxin toxicity. Because digoxin is a drug with a narrow therapeutic window, patients should be advised to avoid taking any of the abovementioned herbs to avoid toxicity.

DIGOXIN—GINSENG (*ELEUTHEROCOCCUS SENTICOSUS*/SIBERIAN GINSENG)

Rating 1

NOTE: *This interaction regards an interference with a diagnostic test, not a true drug interaction.*

Interaction Summary

So-called Siberian ginseng (actually the unrelated herb, *Eleutherococcus senticosus*) has been shown to falsely elevate measured serum digoxin levels without concomitant digoxin toxicity. Thus this is not actually an interaction with the drug but with the *test* for the drug.

Discussion

A 74-year-old man taking digoxin, 0.25 mg orally daily, for atrial fibrillation had been in stable condition for 10 years at a level of 0.9 to 2.2 nmol/L (normal range: 0.6 to 2.6 nmol/L).[1] A routine digoxin measurement was 5.2 nmol/L, but the patient reported no symptoms of digoxin toxicity such as nausea, vomiting, or abnormal vision. His potassium levels, creatinine, and blood urea nitrogen levels were all within the normal range (4.9 mmol/L, 100 μmol/L, and 5.9 mmol/L, respectively). Despite digoxin discontinuation, the level was 4.0 nmol/L on day 28. On

---

Rating Scale:

(1) Significant interaction

(2) Possibly significant interaction

(3) Interaction of relatively little significance

(4) Reported interaction that does not, in fact, exist or is insignificant

day 26 it was discovered that the patient had been taking *Eleutherococcus* ginseng for several months. On discontinuation of the ginseng product, the digoxin level dropped, and when within the normal range, digoxin therapy was resumed. The patient initiated rechallenge with a subsequent increase in digoxin levels without accompanying symptoms of toxicity. The herb capsules were analyzed and were found not to be contaminated with digoxin or digitoxin. *Eleutherococcus* contains eleuthoerosides (not ginsenosides), some of which are chemically similar to the cardiac glycosides of digoxin. Because the patient had no symptoms of toxicity, apparently the herb interfered with the digoxin assay rather than the digoxin itself.

Management Suggestions

Digoxin has a narrow therapeutic window requiring close monitoring with blood assays. *Eleutherococcus* might interfere with this assay and hence presents a practical problem if taken concomitantly with digoxin.

DIGOXIN—KYUSHIN

Rating 2

NOTE: This interaction regards an interference with a diagnostic test, not a true drug interaction.

Interaction Summary

Kyushin may interfere with digoxin assays, creating falsely elevated readings.

Discussion

Kyushin is the dried venom of the Chinese toad *Bufo bufo gargarizans* Cantor, which purportedly has digoxin-like actions.[1] A patient taking digoxin, 0.25 mg/day, for congestive heart failure had a digoxin level of 2.5 mmol/L but no symptoms of digoxin intoxication.[2] The patient was also taking kyushin. On further investigation, it was found that one kyushin tablet had digoxin-like immunoreactivity equivalent to 1.9 μg (TDX analyzer, Abbott Laboratories, North Chicago, IL) and 72 μg of digoxin (Enymun-Test, Boehringer, Mannheim, Germany). Hence, kyushin use may cause spuriously high digoxin levels.

Management Suggestions

Patients should be advised that if they take kyushin while also taking digoxin, accurate measurement of their digoxin levels will be difficult, if not impossible, because of interference with

---

Rating Scale:

(1) Significant interaction

(2) Possibly significant interaction

(3) Interaction of relatively little significance

(4) Reported interaction that does not, in fact, exist or is insignificant

the assay. Because the half-life of kyushin's active ingredients in this respect is unknown, it is not possible to make a recommendation regarding an adequate period of time of kyushin discontinuation before obtaining digoxin assays.

DIGOXIN—LICORICE

Rating 2

OTHER POTENTIALLY IMPLICATED HERBS

If overused as laxative
  Cascara sagrada
  Drug aloe

Senna

Interaction Summary

Licorice may cause a significant decrease in serum potassium, predisposing patients to symptoms of digoxin toxicity.

Discussion

When taken in sufficient doses, licorice can cause hyper-mineralocorticoidism (see the **Spironolactone—Licorice** article).[1] This effect is secondary to the glycyrrhetinic acid content that affects renal tubule potassium secretion, which continues abnormally despite subnormal plasma potassium levels.[2] Clinical manifestations include polyuria, lethargy, paresthesias, muscle cramps, headaches, tetany, peripheral edema, breathlessness, hypertension, and proximal myopathy.[1]

A 51-year-old white man was hospitalized with persistent hypokalemia ranging from 2.3 to 2.9 mEq/L that was determined to be secondary to daily licorice intake of 70 g for 2 months.[3]

Rating Scale:
(1) Significant interaction
(2) Possibly significant interaction

(3) Interaction of relatively little significance
(4) Reported interaction that does not, in fact, exist or is insignificant

Within 1 week of discontinuation, the patient's serum potassium levels were within normal limits.

Two additional cases were reported in a 21-year-old woman and a 35-year-old woman who had daily ingested 120 mg and 50 mg glycyrrhizinic acid, respectively.[4] The patients had potassium levels of 2.6 mmol/L and 2.2 mmol/L (normal: 3.8 to 5.0), respectively. Within 3 weeks of discontinuation, the patients' potassium levels had returned to normal.

Hypokalemia associated with licorice use can be profound, resulting in myopathy, paresthesias, and quadriparesis. This occurred in a 35-year-old man who ingested 20 to 40 g of pure licorice daily for 2 years. He was hospitalized because of rapid-onset flaccid quadriparesis with areflexia and paresthesias. Neurologic examination revealed complete paralysis of proximal muscles of the arms and shoulder girdles, along with weakness of muscles of the forearms and hands, weakness of proximal leg muscles, and moderate weakness of the posterior and anterior neck muscles.[5] His serum potassium level was 2.1 mEq/L.

One often unrecognized source of licorice is chewing tobacco, which resulted in a serum potassium level of 1.8 mmol/L in an 85-year-old man who had ingested 85 g of chewing tobacco daily for 50 years.[6]

Such profound hypokalemia can adversely affect a patient taking digoxin. These patients will be predisposed to digoxin toxicity, which may manifest as anorexia, nausea, vomiting, diarrhea, weakness, visual disturbances (e.g., blurred vision), ventricular tachycardia, and unifocal or multiform premature ventricular contractions.

Management Suggestions

Patients taking digoxin should be advised against using licorice. The potential for hypokalemia should be explained to them in terms of digoxin toxicity. Close monitoring of potassium levels is advised if concomitant licorice use is suspected in a patient prescribed digoxin.

DIGOXIN—MAGNESIUM

Rating 3

RELATED DRUGS

Deslanoside   Digitoxin
Digitalis

Interaction Summary

Magnesium supplements might impair digoxin absorption. However, magnesium deficiency can increase the risk of digoxin toxicity.

Discussion

Magnesium supplementation may be advisable during digoxin treatment, because hypomagnesemia in individuals on digoxin is relatively common and might predispose them to digitalis-induced cardiac arrhythmias.[1-4]

However, taking a magnesium supplement concurrently with digoxin might interfere with the absorption of the drug. Brown and Juhl[5] found that antacids containing magnesium hydroxide, and particularly magnesium trisilicate, substantially reduced digoxin absorption. Physical adsorption of digoxin by the antacids in the GI tract appeared to be the primary mechanism of this interaction.

Rating Scale:
(1) Significant interaction
(2) Possibly significant interaction

(3) Interaction of relatively little significance
(4) Reported interaction that does not, in fact, exist or is insignificant

Later studies, however, found no change in digoxin absorption attributable to magnesium trisilicate.[6] In vitro studies suggest that magnesium carbonate only weakly impairs digoxin absorption.[7] The in vitro model involved absorption across a physiologic membrane that has been shown to correlate well with the in vivo environment.[8]

Management Suggestions

Patients taking digoxin may also need magnesium supplementation. Measurement of serum magnesium levels may be helpful, although they may not accurately reflect tissue levels. Because some evidence indicates that magnesium-containing antacids can impair digoxin absorption, administer digoxin and magnesium supplements at least 2 hours apart.

DIGOXIN—ST. JOHN'S WORT

Rating 1

RELATED DRUGS

Cyclosporine
Indinavir

Oral contraceptives
(possibly)

Interaction Summary

St. John's wort may reduce serum levels of digoxin by interfering with its intestinal absorption.

Discussion

In a single-blind, placebo-controlled study enrolling 25 individuals, St. John's wort significantly reduced serum digoxin levels.[1] The study design involved a 5-day pretreatment with digoxin followed by a 10-day treatment with St. John's wort or placebo. Significant reductions were seen in serum drug trough levels, as well as AUC and C_{max}. These effects were more pronounced the longer the herb was taken.

The lack of change in $t_{1/2}$ for terminal elimination of digoxin led the authors to conclude that the mechanism of interaction was not increased digoxin metabolism but rather due to impaired digoxin absorption or distribution. St. John's wort is thought to induce the activity of an intestinal drug efflux pump

Rating Scale:
(1) Significant interaction
(2) Possibly significant
    interaction

(3) Interaction of relatively little
    significance
(4) Reported interaction that
    does not, in fact, exist or is
    insignificant

called p-glycoprotein (also known as MDR1 or the multidrug-resistance gene).[2,3] P-glycoprotein is a broad-specificity organic drug efflux pump that counteracts intestinal drug absorption and/or enhances renal drug excretion and commonly is induced by agents that also induce CYP3A4 activity[4]; however, digoxin is not metabolized extensively by this cytochrome P-450 isoform. Instead, the authors purport that increased activity of the p-glycoprotein transporter would cause digoxin to be excreted actively into the intestinal lumen instead of being absorbed into the blood supply of intestinal microvilli.

Management Suggestions

Individuals taking digoxin should have serum levels measured if St. John's wort is taken concurrently. Furthermore, if an individual taking both St. John's wort and digoxin discontinues the herb, rebound toxicity may occur. Many patients will not voluntarily admit use of herbs unless questioned directly.

ESTROGEN—BORON

RELATED DRUGS

Conjugated estrogens
Esterified estrogens
Estradiol

Estropipate
Ethinyl estradiol

Interaction Summary

Boron may increase serum levels of endogenous estrogen and minimize the loss of minerals needed for bone mineralization. However, this combination may also increase the risk of estrogen side effects.

Discussion

A single-blind, placebo-controlled, crossover trial found that boron supplementation increased estradiol levels. Eight healthy men took 10 mg/day of supplemental boron for 4 weeks and then took placebo for 4 weeks, or vice versa. The treated group showed significantly increased plasma estradiol and a trend toward increased testosterone levels.[1]

In another study, 12 postmenopausal women received a boron supplement at 3 mg/day, a nutritional dose, after consuming a

---

Rating Scale:
(1) Significant interaction
(2) Possibly significant interaction

(3) Interaction of relatively little significance
(4) Reported interaction that does not, in fact, exist or is insignificant

known daily amount of dietary boron (0.25 mg) for 119 days.[2] Boron supplementation markedly increased serum concentrations of 17-beta-estradiol, the most biologically active form of endogenous human estrogen, as well as testosterone. Additionally, boron supplementation substantially decreased the urinary excretion of calcium.

These findings suggest that, in postmenopausal women consuming a low-boron diet, supplemental boron in amounts commonly found in diets high in fruits and vegetables may help prevent bone demineralization and osteoporosis. However, boron supplementation also presents the potential to increase estrogen-related risks and side effects, such as thromboembolism and breast and uterine cancer.

Management Suggestions

Women receiving ERT or HRT should use boron with caution. If supplementation is desired, it might be advisable to do so by means of a diet high in fruits and vegetables.

ESTROGEN—DONG QUAI

RELATED DRUGS

Conjugated estrogens
Esterified estrogens
Estradiol

Estropipate
Ethinyl estradiol

Interaction Summary

Based on presently available data, it appears unlikely that dong quai will interact with estrogen or estrogen-related entities.

Discussion

Dong quai *(Radix Angelica sinensis)* contains beta-sitosterol, a phytoestrogen.[1] However, in a study of 71 postmenopausal women, transvaginal ultrasonography measuring endometrial thickness, vaginal cell evaluation of cellular maturation, review of Kupperman index for menopausal symptoms, and a diary of vasomotor flushes revealed no estrogen-like responses associated with dong quai.[2]

Hence, apparently the reported beneficial effect of dong quai during menopause cannot be explained in terms of estrogen-like activity. Based on these data, adverse additive or synergistic

---

Rating Scale:

(1) Significant interaction
(2) Possibly significant interaction

(3) Interaction of relatively little significance
(4) Reported interaction that does not, in fact, exist or is insignificant

effects would not be expected if coadministered with estrogen replacement therapy or other similar products.

Management Suggestions

It is unlikely that dosage adjustments will be necessary when these two entities are used together.

ESTROGEN—GINSENG (PANAX GINSENG)

Rating 3

RELATED DRUGS

Conjugated estrogens
Esterified estrogens
Estradiol

Estropipate
Ethinyl estradiol

Interaction Summary

Ginseng reportedly can occasionally cause symptoms of estrogen excess, such as mastalgia, vaginal breakthrough bleeding, nausea, and bloating.

Discussion

Despite a substantial body of animal and human research, no evidence indicates that ginseng ordinarily produces an estrogenic effect. However, several case reports have linked ginseng to symptoms of estrogen excess.

A 70-year-old woman experienced swollen, tender breasts with diffuse nodularity after 3 weeks of ginseng powder administration.[1] These symptoms resolved on discontinuation of ginseng

---

Rating Scale:

(1) Significant interaction
(2) Possibly significant interaction

(3) Interaction of relatively little significance
(4) Reported interaction that does not, in fact, exist or is insignificant

but resumed in two subsequent rechallenges. Serum prolactin levels measured both when the patient was and was not taking ginseng were within the normal range.

In another case report, a 62-year-old woman who had never taken estrogens had a vaginal smear demonstrating a strong estrogenic effect with a maturation index of 0/65/35 (parabasal/intermediate/superficial cells). She had been taking ginseng for 2 weeks.[2]

Vaginal bleeding was also reported in a 72-year-old woman after daily oral administration of 200 mg of ginseng and in another woman after the use of ginseng facial cream.[3,4] In the latter report, a 44-year-old woman experienced abnormal bleeding despite onset of menopause at age 42 years.[4] She was using Fang ginseng face cream (Shanghai, China). Her follicle-stimulating hormone (FSH) level was 36 mIU at this time but increased to 70 mIU 1 month following discontinuation. When she initiated rechallenge, she experienced another episode of uterine bleeding within 1 month with an associated FSH level of 27 mIU. She has had no further episodes of uterine bleeding since ultimately discontinuing use of the facial cream. Although there are no accompanying pharmacokinetics studies, presumably sufficient absorption occurs following dermal use to exert systemic side effects. However, because many Chinese herbal preparations have been found to be contaminated with pharmaceuticals,[5] possibly another explanation exists for these effects.

Management Suggestions

Although it is premature to warn patients against combining ginseng with estrogen medications, the possibility of an interaction should be considered.

ESTROGEN—IPRIFLAVONE

Rating 2

RELATED DRUGS

Conjugated estrogens
Esterified estrogens
Estradiol

Estropipate
Ethinyl estradiol

Interaction Summary

Ipriflavone, a synthetic isoflavone that inhibits bone resorption, may enhance the bone-preserving effects of estrogen as well as provide a benefit when used alone. Combination treatment with estrogen and ipriflavone raises at least some concern that ipriflavone might increase the risk of hormone-dependent uterine and breast malignancies.

Discussion

Agnusdei et al.[1] found that combination treatment with low doses of conjugated estrogen (0.3 mg/day) and ipriflavone (600 mg/day) resulted in a significant increase in forearm bone density after 1 year of treatment (+5.6%; $P = 0.01$) compared to placebo (–1.7%) and conjugated estrogen alone (–1.4%). The authors suggest that a lower dose of estrogen can reduce climacteric symptoms of menopause and prevent uterine atrophy, whereas the addition of ipriflavone provides protection from osteoporosis.

Rating Scale:

(1) Significant interaction
(2) Possibly significant interaction

(3) Interaction of relatively little significance
(4) Reported interaction that does not, in fact, exist or is insignificant

A Korean study focused on differences among treatment with ipriflavone alone, hormone replacement therapy alone, and a combination of the two.[2] After 1 year the bone mineral density of the spine had increased 1% in the ipriflavone group and 3% in the combination ipriflavone and hormone replacement therapy group. The group receiving hormone replacement therapy alone showed a decrease in bone mineral density compared to baseline values.

Another study compared the administration of ipriflavone alone or in combination with low-dose estrogen replacement therapy versus high-dose estrogen replacement therapy.[3] Results demonstrated that lumbar bone mineral density increased with ipriflavone and with high-dose transdermal 17-beta-estradiol, but that the combination of low-dose estrogen and ipriflavone did not yield a gain in bone mineral density.

Gambacciani et al.[4] evaluated the use of 600 mg/day of ipriflavone plus 500 mg of calcium versus 400 mg/day of ipriflavone plus 0.30 mg of conjugated equine estrogens and 500 mg of calcium. These combinations were equally effective, whereas the control (500-mg calcium) or conjugated estrogen alone (0.30 mg) groups showed a comparable rate of loss of bone mineral density. A similar study assessed the effectiveness of ipriflavone plus low doses of conjugated estrogens (0.15 mg/day or 0.30 mg/day). Bone mineral density increased 5.6% at the distal radius in the ipriflavone plus 0.30-mg/day conjugated estrogens group versus 5% in the ipriflavone plus 0.15-mg/day group.[5] In contrast, over the same 12-month period, control groups lost bone mineral density at –1.7% for estrogen alone and –1.4% for placebo.

Nozaki et al.[6] conducted a study in 116 oophorectomized women divided into four groups according to whether they took conjugated equine estrogen, 0.625 mg ($n = 29$); ipriflavone, 600 mg/day ($n = 30$); a combination of conjugated equine estrogen, 0.625 mg/day plus ipriflavone, 600 mg/day ($n = 27$); or placebo ($n = 30$).[6] After 48 weeks, bone mineral density was reduced by 6.1% in the placebo group, by 5.1% in ipriflavone group, by

3.9% in the estrogen group, but by only 1.2% in the group taking both estrogen and ipriflavone.

A study of 79 postmenopausal women with established osteoporosis compared the effects of ipriflavone, ipriflavone plus estriol (1 mg/day), and no treatment on bone mineral density.[7] After 1 year, a time when 4% to 5% decreases in bone mineral density occurred in controls, both treatments were found to prevent loss of bone density as measured at the second metacarpal in the forearm. There were no significant differences between the two treatment groups ($P > 0.1$), suggesting that ipriflavone alone exerts a benefit.

As noted, combination treatment with ipriflavone and estrogens has been advocated to enhance the effects of estrogen on bone tissue. However, findings in some studies raise potential safety concerns. Although ipriflavone by itself has no effect on estrogen-sensitive tissues outside bone, it may potentiate the effects of estrogen on reproductive tissue, specifically the uterus.[8-10] For this reason, HRT is preferable to ERT when such combination treatment is considered. The finding that such potentiation is possible also suggests that an increased risk of hormone-dependent breast malignancies may exist with combination therapy, but thus far this potential risk has not been evaluated.

Management Suggestions

Adding ipriflavone to conventional estrogen therapy for osteoporosis prevention or treatment may produce an additive benefit and also allow lower doses of estrogen to be used, although attention should be paid to the possibility that ipriflavone might increase the risk of hormone-dependent uterine and breast malignancies.

ESTROGEN—RESVERATROL

Rating 3

RELATED DRUGS

Conjugated estrogens   Estropipate
Esterified estrogens   Ethinyl estradiol
Estradiol

Interaction Summary

The supplement resveratrol, marketed as a chemopreventive agent, is closely related chemically to diethylstilbestrol. This has raised concerns of possible interactions between resveratrol and estrogen therapy.

Discussion

In vitro evidence suggests that resveratrol competes at the estrogen receptor with estradiol, activating estrogen-responsive reporter genes, and stimulating proliferation of estrogen-dependent T47D breast cancer cells.[1]

Management Suggestions

Individuals taking estrogen should avoid resveratrol supplements.

Rating Scale:
(1) Significant interaction
(2) Possibly significant interaction
(3) Interaction of relatively little significance
(4) Reported interaction that does not, in fact, exist or is insignificant

ETOPOSIDE—ST. JOHN'S WORT

Rating 2

RELATED DRUGS

Doxorubicin   Teniposide

Mitoxantrone

Interaction Summary

A component of St. John's wort (hypericin) may interfere with the desired anticancer action of etoposide.

Discussion

Etoposide and related drugs are useful anticancer agents for treatment of breast, prostate, lung, and colon cancers, as well as some types of leukemia. These drugs work by trapping topoisomerase II (an enzyme essential to cancer cell growth) onto DNA, thereby triggering cancer cell death.

An in vitro assay using purified human topoisomerase II found that hypericin from St. John's wort can reverse the topoisomerase II–poisoning effect of etoposide.[1] This effect was quite potent, with hypericin completely reversing topoisomerase II–DNA complexes at one third the concentration of etoposide.[2] However, these investigators have yet to determine the effect of hypericin on the anticancer action of etoposide in intact tumor cells.

Rating Scale:

(1) Significant interaction

(2) Possibly significant interaction

(3) Interaction of relatively little significance

(4) Reported interaction that does not, in fact, exist or is insignificant

Management Suggestions

Although it is difficult to extrapolate from the in vitro data to humans, it would be prudent for cancer patients to avoid St. John's wort while on any chemotherapeutic regimen containing a topoisomerase II–poisoning drug such as etoposide until more extensive studies are completed.

Although some newer St. John's wort products are being manufactured free of hypericin to reduce side effects, such products still may be problematic. Etoposide can be exported from tumor cells by p-glycoprotein and inactivated by CYP3A4[3]; both of these processes may be induced by St. John's wort (see the **Cyclosporine—St. John's Wort, Indinavir—St. John's Wort,** and **Digoxin—St. John's Wort** articles), but this effect has not been specifically tied to hypericin.

FEXOFENADINE—FRUIT JUICE

Rating 3

Interaction Summary

Grapefruit, orange, and apple juice may reduce the efficacy of fexofenadine (Allegra).

Discussion

Fexofenadine is a substrate for organic anion–transporting polypeptide (OATP) and p-glycoprotein. A study suggests that grapefruit, orange, and apple juice inhibit intestinal uptake of fexofenadine through interactions with OATP and p-glycoprotein.[1]

Management Suggestions

Individuals using fexofenadine should be informed that increased consumption of fruit juice might decrease the effectiveness of the medication.

Rating Scale:
(1) Significant interaction
(2) Possibly significant interaction

(3) Interaction of relatively little significance
(4) Reported interaction that does not, in fact, exist or is insignificant

FLUOROQUINOLONES—
MINERALS

Rating 2

RELATED DRUGS

Ciprofloxacin   Norfloxacin
Enoxacin   Ofloxacin
Grepafloxacin   Sparfloxacin
Lomefloxacin   Trovafloxacin

OTHER POTENTIALLY IMPLICATED SUPPLEMENTS

Aluminum   Magnesium
Calcium   Zinc
Iron

Interaction Summary

The minerals calcium, iron, and zinc may interfere with the absorption of fluoroquinolone antibiotics. Antacids containing aluminum and magnesium may interact similarly with these antibiotics.

Discussion

Calcium-containing dairy products or calcium-containing antacids may decrease the absorption of some fluoroquinolones. Milk (200 ml, providing 218 mg of calcium) reduced the absorp-

Rating Scale:
(1) Significant interaction
(2) Possibly significant
    interaction

(3) Interaction of relatively little
    significance
(4) Reported interaction that
    does not, in fact, exist or is
    insignificant

tion of norfloxacin and ciprofloxacin in six fasted volunteers.[1,2] Norfloxacin bioavailability (AUC) was reduced by 38% compared to an antibiotic-water combination. In seven volunteers, milk and yogurt decreased the bioavailability of ciprofloxacin by 30% and 36%, respectively.[2] In contrast, milk had no effect on the bioavailability of lomefloxacin[3] or ofloxacin.[4]

Calcium carbonate–containing antacids reduced norfloxacin bioavailability by 38% but had no effect on lomefloxacin[3] or ofloxacin.[5]

Iron may form a complex with some fluoroquinolones and decrease their absorption. Ferrous sulfate, 325 mg, decreased the bioavailability of ciprofloxacin, 500 mg, by 64%.[6] A crossover study of eight volunteers found that giving ciprofloxacin with ferrous sulfate, 300 mg, ferrous gluconate, 600 mg, or a combination tablet containing 10 mg of elemental iron reduced the bioavailability of the antibiotic by 46%, 67%, and 57%, respectively.[7] Similar results were found when ferrous sulfate was given with norfloxacin[8] and ofloxacin.[9] Sustained-release ferrous sulfate produced clinically insignificant effects on ofloxacin and lomefloxacin.[3,10]

Zinc may decrease the absorption of some fluoroquinolones. A crossover study of 12 volunteers found that a multivitamin containing zinc reduced ciprofloxacin bioavailability by 24%.[6] Another study of eight volunteers found that zinc sulfate, 200 mg, significantly decreased the bioavailability of norfloxacin.[8]

Most studies have found that antacids containing aluminum and magnesium markedly reduced the bioavailability of fluoroquinolones, including ciprofloxacin,[10] norfloxacin,[11] enoxacin,[12] lomefloxacin,[13] and trovafloxacin.[14] Aluminum hydroxide was reported to reduce the bioavailability of levofloxacin and sparfloxacin by 45% and 35%, respectively.[15]

Management Suggestions

Give mineral supplements and milk as far apart as possible from fluoroquinolone antibiotics. Administer antacids at least 6 hours before or 2 hours after fluoroquinolone antibiotics.

FOLATE—ALUMINUM HYDROXIDE

Interaction Summary

Antacids containing aluminum hydroxide may bind to folate and reduce its absorption.

Discussion

Adequate folate nurture is essential for the prevention of numerous illnesses, including heart disease and neural tube defect. However, folic acid deficiency is common in developed countries.[1] For this reason, drugs that impair folate absorption, even slightly, may present a real health risk. Antacids containing aluminum hydroxide may fall into this category.

Folate absorption is maximal in the jejunum, where the influence of gastric acid provides ideal conditions, and alkalinization of the proximal small intestine has been found to diminish folate absorption.[2]

A commonly used antacid (aluminum and magnesium hydroxide) did indeed reduce folate absorption to a small extent, apparently not by its effect on stomach acid but by adsorbing the vitamin.[3] To examine the effect of the antacid on dietary folate absorption, researchers gave the antacid to 30 participants, 1 hour and 3 hours after consuming a specially formulated

Rating Scale:
(1) Significant interaction
(2) Possibly significant interaction

(3) Interaction of relatively little significance
(4) Reported interaction that does not, in fact, exist or is insignificant

liquid meal containing 200 μg of folate. The results showed that folate absorption was 50.6% with the formula meal alone compared to 43.1% when the antacid was given after the formula meal.

Surprisingly, the decrease in folate absorption could not be accounted for by the reduction of peptic acidity associated with an antacid, as would be expected. Monitoring of pH values at the ligament of Treitz showed that acidity actually increased slightly during the 2-hour period after the liquid meal despite the influence of the antacid.

Subsequent in vitro studies found that the aluminum hydroxide component of the antacid physically attached to folate. Aluminum hydroxide is present as a gel over a pH range of approximately 3.7 to 10.[4] As the pH of the solution increases, removal of folate commences at a pH just below 4.0, when the hydroxide begins to precipitate. It is probable that the gel adsorbs folate onto its surface and then takes it out of contact with the aqueous phase as gel particles agglomerate. The effect on folate absorption was minor, and this interaction may be clinically important only in individuals who take antacids regularly and whose diets are marginal in folate.

Management Suggestions

Antacid-induced reduction in folate absorption appears to be small. However, because folate deficiency is common, individuals who regularly take aluminum hydroxide antacids might be advised to take a folate supplement on general principles.

FOLATE—CARBAMAZEPINE

Rating 2

RELATED DRUGS

Barbiturates	Primidone
Phenobarbital	Valproic acid

Interaction Summary

The anticonvulsants carbamazepine, phenobarbital, and primidone may lower serum folate levels by both increasing its hepatic metabolism and decreasing its absorption. Primidone, which is metabolized to phenobarbital, may also inhibit the growth of folate-dependent microorganisms. Valproic acid appears not to induce enzymes but may decrease folate absorption.

Discussion

Adequate folate nutriture is essential for the prevention of numerous illnesses, including heart disease and neural tube defect. However, folic acid deficiency is common in developed countries.[1] For this reason, drugs that impair folate absorption, even slightly, may present a real health risk. Anticonvulsants are believed to fall into this category.

Folate deficiency occurs in some epileptic patients taking anticonvulsant drugs, and is a high incidence of neuropsychiatric

Rating Scale:
(1) Significant interaction
(2) Possibly significant interaction

(3) Interaction of relatively little significance
(4) Reported interaction that does not, in fact, exist or is insignificant

illness occurs in cases of megaloblastic anemia caused by folate deficiency.[2]

Kishi et al.[3] measured serum folate concentrations in age-matched control subjects without anemia and in epileptic outpatients being treated with a single anticonvulsant drug, including carbamazepine, phenobarbital, and valproate. A protein-binding radioassay was used to demonstrate that reduced serum folate was associated with hepatic enzyme induction by carbamazepine and phenobarbital, but not valproate, compared to controls. Primidone, which is metabolized to phenobarbital, would be expected to have similar effects. Additionally, primidone has been found to inhibit the growth of folate-dependent microorganisms.[4] Valproate was not associated with enzyme induction and did not reduce serum folate levels significantly. An earlier study confirmed valproate's lack of enzyme-inducing effects. Folate absorption was measured in five patients prior to and after 2 months of valproate or carbamazepine therapy. Although valproate had no enzyme-inducing effect, it did interfere with folate absorption as indicated by depressed plasma folate concentrations with no accompanying increase in renal clearance.[5] Carbamazepine similarly interfered with folate absorption but curiously had no apparent effect on hepatic metabolism in this study, even though it is categorized as an enzyme inducer.

Isojarvi et al.[6] demonstrated ability of carbamazepine to increase the hepatic metabolism of folate without measuring serum folate levels. Researchers monitored 25 patients with epilepsy for 5 years after they started carbamazepine. To further clarify the effects of carbamazepine in 12 patients, carbamazepine was replaced with oxcarbazepine, a derivative of carbamazepine but without its liver enzyme–inducing properties. Carbamazepine therapy altered gamma-glutamyl transferase (GGT) activity and several hematologic parameters: it decreased WBC and RBC counts and increased mean corpuscular volume (MCV) and serum GGT activity. The increased MCV indicated macrocytosis, but this was not associated with anemia. Replacing carbamazepine with oxcarbazepine tended to reverse these abnormalities: WBC and MCV counts normalized; serum GGT activity decreased along with increases in erythrocyte folate concentrations and serum vitamin B_{12} levels. All of these indicate a normalization of the liver CYP450 enzyme system formerly induced by carbamazepine.

Of 62 patients with epilepsy studied by Reynolds et al.,[7] 54 were taking phenobarbital, primidone, or phenytoin singly or in various combinations, with 8 serving as untreated controls. Serum folate concentrations in 76% of treated patients were below the range found in control subjects, and average folate concentration for the treated patients was 3.7 ng/ml compared to 6.4 ng/ml for the controls. A folate deficiency usually is defined as less than 3 ng/ml (7 nmol/L).[8] None of the treated patients was anemic, but 17 of 45 in whom bone marrow was examined showed megaloblastic hemopoiesis. Only 7 of the 54 treated patients showed macrocytosis.

Anticonvulsant-induced low serum folate levels can cause elevated homocysteine levels, which is believed to increase the risk of atherosclerosis. Ono et al.[2] evaluated 130 epileptic patients taking anticonvulsant single-drug or multidrug therapy (including carbamazepine) compared to 81 control subjects. Low serum folate levels correlated with high serum homocysteine levels. Of the four folate-deficient patients, all had received long-term (>7 years) multidrug therapy. Folate therapy normalized their homocysteine and folate levels. Measuring folate and homocysteine levels may be beneficial in patients taking anticonvulsants, especially those on long-term multidrug therapy.

Because carbamazepine and other anticonvulsant drugs deplete folate, babies born to anticonvulsant users are at increased risk for neural tube birth defects such as spina bifida and anencephaly. Folate is believed to be a cofactor in the metabolism of carbamazepine and several other anticonvulsant drugs. Inadequate folate may prevent complete carbamazepine metabolism and cause the accumulation of intermediate epoxides that may contribute to the fetal abnormalities observed with anticonvulsant therapy.[9]

One study compared mothers receiving anticonvulsants including carbamazepine, usually combined with other anticonvulsant therapy (e.g., phenytoin, phenobarbital), with and without folate supplementation.[10] In 24 women not receiving folate—the retrospective part of the study—the frequency of congenital malformations among the 66 newborns was 15% (10 children); 3 of the 10 were stillborn or died immediately after delivery. In the 22 women receiving folate—the prospective part of the study—all 33 infants were born alive and no congenital malformations occurred.

Carbamazepine and other anticonvulsants also may have a direct role in teratogenesis, according to a review of studies by Lewis et al.[9] Women with epilepsy who are contemplating pregnancy should be treated with the fewest folate-lowering drugs possible and should receive folate supplementation.

Since 1998 the FDA has required that grain products such as cereals be fortified with folic acid in such a way as to increase actual daily intake of folic acid by approximately 78 µg.[11] Researchers predict that this dietary folate fortification will have a significant, although not optimal, effect in preventing neural tube birth defects. The current FDA recommendation is that all women of childbearing age receive at least 400 µg of folate daily before and during pregnancy to prevent these types of complications, but that does not take into account women on anticonvulsant drugs.

Management Suggestions

Folate supplementation may prevent anticonvulsant-induced folate depletion. A comprehensive multivitamin supplement, which might typically provide 400 µg of folate and 6 µg of vitamin B_{12}, may be sufficient, but a higher folate dose may be needed in some cases, especially with anticonvulsant polytherapy.[12] Because it has been suggested that the action of anticonvulsant drugs may be at least in part related to their folate-reducing effects, it may be desirable to administer enough folate to prevent a deficiency, but not an excessive amount.

FOLATE—CIMETIDINE

Rating 3

RELATED DRUGS

Famotidine	Omeprazole
Lansoprazole	Rabeprazole sodium
Nizatidine	Ranitidine

Interaction Summary

By reducing stomach acid, H_2 antagonists and proton pump inhibitors may marginally reduce the body's absorption of folate.

Discussion

Adequate folate nutriture is essential for the prevention of numerous illnesses, including heart disease and neural tube defects. However, folic acid deficiency is common in developed countries.[1] For this reason, drugs that impair folate absorption, even slightly, may present a real health risk. H_2 antagonists and proton pump inhibitors may fall in this category.

Folate absorption is maximal in the jejunum, where the influence of gastric acid provides the ideal conditions, and alkalinization of the proximal small intestine has been found to diminish folate absorption.[2]

Rating Scale:

(1) Significant interaction

(2) Possibly significant interaction

(3) Interaction of relatively little significance

(4) Reported interaction that does not, in fact, exist or is insignificant

The H_2 antagonists cimetidine and ranitidine have been found to reduce folate absorption to a small extent.[3] Proton pump inhibitors might be expected to have a similar effect.

To examine the effect of histamine H_2 antagonists on dietary folate absorption, 30 participants followed a standard regimen of either cimetidine or ranitidine and then were fed a specially formulated liquid meal containing 200 μg of folate. Folate absorption was 50% with the formula meal alone compared to 45.8% with the formula meal plus cimetidine. Ranitidine also reduced folate absorption, but the change was not statistically significant.

Monitoring of pH values at the ligament of Treitz showed that the slight acidity existing before consumption of the liquid meal was generally maintained during the 2-hour period after the meal.

In vitro studies conducted in association with this trial found that neither cimetidine nor ranitidine physically bound folate or interfered with its metabolism (there was no inhibition of dihydrofolate reductase at concentrations of 5 and 50 μmol/L). The interaction might therefore be attributed to the ability of the drugs to prevent a decrease in intestinal pH, which would have favored folate absorption. Curiously, cimetidine reduced folate absorption more than ranitidine even though ranitidine increased intestinal pH the most.

Management Suggestions

The extent of drug-induced folate absorption appears to be relatively small, but patients receiving long-term therapy with an H_2 antagonist or a proton pump inhibitor may benefit from folate supplementation.

FOLATE—METHOTREXATE

Rating 1

RELATED DRUGS

Pyrimethamine   Trimetrexate

Interaction Summary

Treatment with methotrexate can impair folate status, and this may cause some of the symptoms of methotrexate toxicity. In certain disease states, folate supplementation has been found to decrease methotrexate toxicity without interfering with its therapeutic effects.

Discussion

Methotrexate is a folate antagonist that reversibly inhibits dihydrofolate reductase, the enzyme that reduces folate to active tetrahydrofolate. The attendant decrease in tetrahydrofolate limits the availability of single-carbon fragments needed in the synthesis of purines, DNA, and cellular proteins. This produces immunosuppressant and antineoplastic effects.

Methotrexate's toxicity is in part related to impaired folate status.[1,2] Folinic acid (leucovorin), a reduced form of folate, has been used to decrease symptoms of methotrexate-induced toxicity such as gastrointestinal intolerance. However, higher doses

---

Rating Scale:

(1) Significant interaction

(2) Possibly significant interaction

(3) Interaction of relatively little significance

(4) Reported interaction that does not, in fact, exist or is insignificant

of folinic acid can reverse the effects of methotrexate therapy, an action used deliberately in the so-called leucovorin rescue.

Folate may be a better choice than folinic acid for minimizing methotrexate side effects. In certain conditions, it has been found to lessen methotrexate toxicity without compromising its effectiveness. The difference is that folinic acid does not require reduction by dihydrofolate reductase.

In a 48-week, double-blind, placebo-controlled trial of 434 individuals with active rheumatoid arthritis, use of folic acid (1 mg/day, doubled when MTX dosage reached 15 mg/week) or folinic acid resulted in reduced toxicity-related discontinuation of MTX due to decreased incidence of elevated liver enzyme levels.[3] MTX dosages were adjusted upward based on symptoms, and slightly higher dosages of MTX were required in the two folate supplementation groups. No improvement was seen in incidence, duration, or severity of other side effects.

One study examined the effect of folate, 5 mg/day, on 78 patients receiving low-dose (2.5 to 30 mg), once-weekly oral methotrexate therapy for psoriasis.[4] Gastrointestinal symptoms were dose related and occurred in 32% of patients. Folate was found to eliminate these symptoms without interfering with the therapeutic effect of methotrexate.

A randomized, double-blind, placebo-controlled study of 79 patients taking low-dose methotrexate therapy for rheumatoid arthritis found similar results.[5] Participants received either 5 mg or 27.5 mg of oral folate therapy weekly or placebo. Methotrexate was started at a median oral dose of 7.5 mg/week and increased in 2.5-mg increments as needed. Folate was given 5 days a week on the days methotrexate was not given. Methotrexate side effects were low (and almost identical) in both folate groups compared to placebo, and neither dose affected methotrexate efficacy.

Another double-blind, placebo-controlled study monitored 75 individuals with rheumatoid arthritis who were already taking methotrexate and folate, 5 mg/day.[6] All were asked to discontinue taking their folate supplements. Half were then given placebo and the other half received folate again. Participants were then monitored for a year. The primary outcome measure was discontinuation of methotrexate usage. The results showed a signficantly greater discontinuation rate in the placebo group (46%) compared to the folate group (21%), suggesting a more severe side effects profile in those taking placebo. Moreover, methotrexate's effects were not significantly blunted by folate.

Folate supplementation also may be appropriate in juvenile rheumatoid arthritis.[7] However, it is possible that folate might interfere with the effectiveness of methotrexate in other disease states.

Management Suggestions

Folate supplementation may be advisable in individuals taking it for rheumatoid arthritis, juvenile rheumatoid arthritis, or psoriasis. For other disease states, caution is advised as inhibition of methotrexate's effectiveness might conceivably occur.

FOLATE—NSAIDs

RELATED DRUGS

Aspirin	Meclofenamate
Bromfenac	Mefenamic acid
Diclofenac	Meloxicam
Etodolac	Nabumetone
Fenoprofen	Naproxen
Flurbiprofen	Oxaprozin
Ibuprofen	Piroxicam
Indomethacin	Sulfasalazine
Ketoprofen	Sulindac
Ketorolac	Tolmetin

Interaction Summary

Nonsteroidal antiinflammatory drugs (NSAIDs) may interfere with folate metabolism.

Discussion

Adequate folate nutriture is essential for the prevention of numerous illnesses, including heart disease and neural tube defect. However, folic acid deficiency is common in developed countries.[1] For this reason, drugs that even slightly impair folate absorption or metabolism may present a real health risk. NSAIDs

---

Rating Scale:

(1) Significant interaction
(2) Possibly significant interaction

(3) Interaction of relatively little significance
(4) Reported interaction that does not, in fact, exist or is insignificant

may fall into this category. Tissue culture experiments have demonstrated that many NSAIDs and NSAID-like drugs are competitive inhibitors of enzymes involved in folate metabolism, including AICAR transformylase and dihydrofolate reductase.[2,3] Among these drugs are aspirin, ibuprofen, indomethacin, mefenamic acid, naproxen, piroxicam, salicylic acid, sulfasalazine, and sulindac.

A drug structure consisting of an aromatic ring with a side chain containing a carboxylic acid group appears to be a requirement for inhibition of the transformylase. Drugs such as piroxicam, with no carboxylic acid group, inhibit dihydrofolate reductase.

One woman was given aspirin, 650 mg orally, every 4 hours for 3 days during an 11-day study.[4] Aspirin induced a significant but reversible decrease in total and bound serum folate and a small but insignificant increase in urinary folate excretion. A follow-up in vitro study reported in the same article found that aspirin significantly displaces bound serum folate.

In a study of 25 outpatients with arthritis treated with sulfasalazine, median serum folate level was significantly lower in the treated group compared to a group of 72 healthy hospital staff.[5] Median tHcy (plasma total homocysteine), a sensitive marker for folate deficiency, was significantly higher in the treated group. Five patients (20%) had tHcy levels exceeding the upper normal limit. In folate deficiency the synthesis of methionine from homocysteine is impaired by the decreased availability of 5-methyltetrahydrofolate, leading to homocysteine accumulation.

Along with effects on folate enzymes, sulfasalazine appears to competitively inhibit intestinal folate transport and absorption, according to a tissue culture study.[6]

Management Suggestions

Monitoring for folate deficiency and increasing dietary folate or giving supplemental folate as needed may be advisable.

FOLATE—ORAL
CONTRACEPTIVES

Rating 4

Interaction Summary

Oral contraceptives (OCs) have been reported to lower serum and/or red blood cell folate in most, but not all, studies. However, this does not appear to cause a folate deficiency under ordinary circumstances.

Discussion

A 1991 study followed 29 women taking OCs containing 30 µg of estrogen over four cycles, with 31 women serving as controls.[1] The results showed that OC treatment did not lower folate levels or induce folate deficiency and that folate supplementation is not routinely required for women during OC use or after its discontinuation.

A 1993 study measured serum folate levels after oral folate loading in 29 users of OCs containing less than 50 µg of estrogen and in 13 women serving as controls.[2] Median serum folate concentrations were decreased in OC users, reaching statistically significant lower levels after 210 minutes (260 nmol/L) compared to controls (400 nmol/L). However, folate deficiency did not occur. Similar results were reported in an observational study of 229 female adolescents taking OCs.[3] Studies involving high-estrogen OCs also have found no evidence of folate deficiency.[2]

Rating Scale:
(1) Significant interaction
(2) Possibly significant interaction
(3) Interaction of relatively little significance
(4) Reported interaction that does not, in fact, exist or is insignificant

Management Suggestions

Although OCs have not been implicated in producing clinically significant folate deficiency, folate deficiency is common in the population at large. Folate supplementation in standard nutritional doses may therefore be beneficial on general principles.

FOLATE—PHENYTOIN

Rating 2

RELATED DRUGS

Ethotoin   Mephenytoin

Interaction Summary

The interaction between phenytoin and folate is dual in effect. Phenytoin decreases serum folate levels, and folate decreases serum phenytoin levels.[1]

Discussion

Adequate folate nutriture is essential for the prevention of numerous illnesses, including heart disease and neural tube defect. However, folate deficiency is common in developed countries.[2] For this reason, drugs that even slightly impair folate absorption may present a real health risk.

Folate deficiency occurs in some patients with epilepsy taking anticonvulsant drugs and there is a high incidence of neuropsychiatric illness in cases of megaloblastic anemia caused by folate deficiency.[3]

The double-edged nature of this interaction is fairly complex. Phenytoin appears to reduce folate absorption by competing

Rating Scale:
(1) Significant interaction
(2) Possibly significant interaction
(3) Interaction of relatively little significance
(4) Reported interaction that does not, in fact, exist or is insignificant

with it for absorption in the small intestine.[4] Additionally, phenytoin induces microsomal oxidase enzymes, which accelerates the metabolic breakdown of folate.[1,5] Anticonvulsant-induced low serum folate levels can cause elevated homocysteine levels, which is believed to increase the risk of atherosclerosis.[3] Ono et al.[3] evaluated 130 epileptic patients taking anticonvulsant monotherapy or polytherapy (including phenytoin) compared to 81 control subjects. Low serum folate levels correlated with high serum homocysteine levels. Of the four folate-deficient patients, all had received long-term (>7 years) polytherapy. Folate therapy returned their homocysteine and folate levels to normal. Measuring folate and homocysteine levels may be beneficial in patients taking anticonvulsants, especially those receiving long-term polytherapy.

Conversely, folate is believed to affect phenytoin levels by its involvement in phenytoin metabolism.[4] Phenytoin and many other anticonvulsants are metabolized to form epoxides. Folate may be a cofactor for the enzyme epoxide hydrolase. High folate levels could therefore accelerate the metabolism of anticonvulsants, and inadequate folate levels could impair their metabolism.[6] In the latter case, incomplete metabolism could allow the accumulation of highly reactive epoxides, which may contribute to the fetal abnormalities observed with anticonvulsant therapy. Furthermore, competition for brain-cell surface receptors may also help explain how high doses of folate (>1 mg daily) can compromise phenytoin seizure control.[4] Folate is associated with a "pseudo–steady state" in which phenytoin appears to be at steady state but is not. Starting phenytoin and folate supplementation together prevents folate depletion and enables phenytoin to achieve steady-state concentrations sooner.

A randomized crossover study of six women of childbearing age illustrates the interdependence of the phenytoin-folate interaction.[4] It consisted of two treatments: treatment 1 was 300 mg of phenytoin daily, and treatment 2 was 300 mg of phenytoin plus 1 mg of folate daily. Dietary folate intake during each treatment was not significantly different. The treatment 1 group showed a 38% reduction in serum folate level with a serum phenytoin concentration in the low therapeutic range. The treatment 2 group showed a 26% increase in serum folate level with a phenytoin level similar to that in treatment 1. Only one woman achieved phenytoin steady state during treatment 1, but four women achieved steady state during treatment 2.

Of the anticonvulsant drugs, hydantoins such as phenytoin are most commonly associated with birth abnormalities.[6] Because phenytoin and other anticonvulsant drugs deplete folate, babies born to anticonvulsant users are at increased risk for neural tube birth defects such as spina bifida and anencephaly. One study compared mothers receiving anticonvulsive therapy with and without folate supplementation.[7] In 24 women not receiving folate—the retrospective part of the study—the frequency of congenital malformations among the 66 newborns was 15% (10 children); 3 of the 10 were stillborn or died immediately after delivery. In the 22 women receiving folate—the prospective part of the study—all 33 infants were born alive and no congenital malformations occurred. Phenytoin and other anticonvulsants may also have a direct role in teratogenesis, according to a review of studies by Lewis et al.[6] Women with epilepsy who are contemplating pregnancy should be treated with the fewest folate-lowering drugs possible and should receive folate supplementation.

Since 1998, the FDA has required that grain products such as cereals be fortified with folic acid, which was expected to increase daily folic acid intake by about 100 μg. To confirm the effect of this folate fortification, researchers had 51 women ages 17 to 40 exclude folic acid–fortified foods (primarily breakfast cereals) from their diet for 12 weeks.[8] All subjects had a normal initial folate status as measured by red blood cell folate concentrations. The result was an average decrease in folate intake by 78 μg daily, which caused a significant reduction in red blood cell folate. This, then, is about the amount of extra folate expected to be provided by the folate fortification requirements. Researchers predict that this dietary folate fortification will have a significant, although not optimal, effect in preventing neural tube birth defects. It is generally recommended that all women of childbearing age consume at least 400 μg of folate daily before and during pregnancy to prevent these types of complications, but that does not take into account women taking anticonvulsant drugs.

Management Suggestions

Folate supplementation may be necessary to prevent phenytoin-induced folate depletion. Starting phenytoin and folate supplementation at the same time appears to neutralize both sides of this interaction.[1] A comprehensive multivitamin supplement, which might typically provide 400 μg of folate and 6 μg of vitamin B_{12}, may be sufficient, but a higher folate dose may be needed in some cases, especially with anticonvulsant polytherapy.[4] Because it has been suggested that the action of anticonvulsant drugs may be at least in part related to their folate-reducing effects, it may be desirable to administer enough folate to prevent a deficiency, but not an excessive amount.

Monitor serum phenytoin levels and clinical effects. Be aware of the possibility of decreased seizure control when folate supplementation is begun or increased phenytoin toxicity when folate supplementation is stopped, and adjust the phenytoin dose as needed.

FOLATE—TRIAMTERENE

Rating 4

Interaction Summary

High-dose triamterene therapy might cause folate deficiency in patients with risk factors for folate depletion.

Discussion

Adequate folate nutriture is essential for the prevention of numerous illnesses, including heart disease and neural tube defect. However, folic acid deficiency is common in developed countries.[1] For this reason, drugs that impair folate absorption, even slightly, may present a real health risk. Triamterene may be implicated when taken at high doses, or in at-risk populations.

Triamterene is a weak folate antagonist because of its structural similarity to folic acid. It could impair both folate absorption as well as the action of dihydrofolate reductase. However, in an observational study of two free-living populations, triamterene was not associated with folate deficiency.[2] One population consisted of 272 elderly individuals not living in institutions who participated in a nutrition survey; 32 were taking triamterene, and 240 were taking other antihypertensive therapy. The dose of triamterene for each subject was not available to researchers, but is believed to be 150 mg/day or less because the drug was taken for conditions other than chronic liver disease and portal hypertension. The other population consisted of 27 individuals

Rating Scale:
(1) Significant interaction
(2) Possibly significant interaction

(3) Interaction of relatively little significance
(4) Reported interaction that does not, in fact, exist or is insignificant

attending a hypertension clinic, including 18 taking triamterene, 50 to 150 mg/day. The findings suggest that chronic triamterene therapy at the doses examined in this study was not associated with indications of folate deficiency. However, because this was an observational study, the possibility of confounding variables is a concern.

In contrast, high-dose triamterene (150 to 600 mg/day) for treatment of ascites in individuals with cirrhosis has been associated with the development of folate-responsive megaloblastic anemia.[3] It is not clear whether the high dosage of triamterene, the liver disease, or the combination was responsible for this effect.

Management Suggestions

Typical triamterene doses in most patients should not significantly affect folate status. However, when high doses are used in individuals with cirrhosis, folate supplementation should be considered. Indeed, because of the prevalence of folate deficiency in the general population, folate supplementation on general principles may be advisable.

FOLATE—TRIMETHOPRIM/ SULFAMETHOXAZOLE

Rating 1

RELATED DRUGS

Dapsone (DDS)   Sulfones
Sulfonamides

Interaction Summary

The drugs trimethoprim (TMP) and sulfamethoxazole (SMZ) may impair folate metabolism to a clinically significant extent. This can be reversed with folate supplementation. However, there are concerns that such supplementation could antagonize the effects of the drug.

Discussion

Adequate folate nutriture is essential for the prevention of numerous illnesses, including heart disease and neural tube defect. However, folate deficiency is common in developed countries.[1] For this reason, drugs that impair folate metabolism, even slightly, may present a real health risk. TMP may fall into this category.

Like its relatives methotrexate and pyrimethamine, TMP is a folate antagonist that inhibits dihydrofolate reductase (DHFR),

---

Rating Scale:
(1) Significant interaction
(2) Possibly significant interaction

(3) Interaction of relatively little significance
(4) Reported interaction that does not, in fact, exist or is insignificant

the enzyme that reduces folic acid to active tetrahydrofolic acid.[2] Sulfonamides such as sulfamethoxazole interfere with folate in a different fashion, competitively displacing PABA from its binding site on an enzyme that catalyzes a key step in the biosynthesis of folic acid.[3] The combined effect may be significant inhibition of folate production. Microorganisms that must synthesize their own folate are susceptible to these antimicrobial drugs; fortunately, bacteria are much more sensitive to the folate-inhibiting action of these agents than are human beings and other mammals. However, there is still some concern that the drugs may interfere with folate status in humans.

One study examined folate metabolism in 10 normal patients treated with TMP (1 g/day) for 4 weeks and 14 patients with chronic genitourinary infections treated with both TMP (1 g/day) and sulfisoxazole for periods up to 2 years.[2] Hematologic changes (e.g., altered plasma and RBC folate levels, high lobe count of granulocytes, formiminoglutamic acid excretion, evidence of megaloblastic hematopoiesis in the marrow) were correlated with inhibition of folate metabolism. Hematologic toxicity was found in four patients, two in each group. In the short-term group, one patient developed thrombocytopenia and another developed anemia associated with transitional megaloblastosis. One patient in the long-term group developed thrombocytopenia and leukopenia, which were reversed by administration of folic acid, 5 mg/day. However, in most cases, a folic acid dose of 400 μg/day was sufficient to ensure hematologic normalcy.

TMP 1 g/day for periods in excess of 14 days appears to impair folate utilization to some extent, and this may lead to mild and folate-reversible hematologic changes. It is possible that high doses of folate might interfere with the antibacterial effects of TMP.

Management Suggestions

Folate supplementation at nutritional doses may be advisable in patients taking these antimicrobial agents for periods exceeding 14 days. If megaloblastic changes occur, discontinuation of the drug and higher folate supplementation may be indicated.

FUROSEMIDE— GINSENG/GERMANIUM

RELATED DRUGS

Bumetanide   Torsemide
Ethacrynic acid

Interaction Summary

Although ginseng itself does not appear to interact with these medications, germanium-supplemented ginseng products reportedly can cause diuretic resistance.

Discussion

Diuretic resistance has been observed in a patient taking germanium-containing ginseng.[1] This 63-year-old man with membranous glomerulonephritis was treated with furosemide and cyclosporine on hospitalization for edema and hypertension (186/100 mm Hg). Ten days before hospitalization, he began to take 10 to 12 tablets daily of a germanium-containing ginseng preparation (Uncle Hsu's Korean ginseng). While hospitalized he did not take this preparation and responded to furosemide 240 mg intravenously every 8 hours. After discharge he resumed the ginseng preparation in conjunction with furosemide 80 mg orally twice daily. Over the ensuing 14 days, edema and hyper-

---

Rating Scale:

(1) Significant interaction

(2) Possibly significant interaction

(3) Interaction of relatively little significance

(4) Reported interaction that does not, in fact, exist or is insignificant

tension worsened despite an increase in furosemide to 240 mg twice daily. Within 48 hours of rehospitalization (with discontinuation of the ginseng product), diuresis became effective.

Patients taking germanium have developed nephrotoxicity with increased concentrations of lipofuscin granules in the cells of the thick ascending limb of the loop of Henle.[2,3] As this is the site of action of furosemide, it was concluded that germanium was instrumental in inducing resistance to furosemide.

Management Suggestions

Patients may elect to take ginseng-germanium combination products in the belief that these lessen their risks of cancer.[4] However, if used together with high-loop diuretics, it is possible that diuretic resistance will ensue. Concomitant use should be avoided.

FUROSEMIDE—GOSSYPOL

Rating 2

RELATED DRUGS

Bumetanide

Ethacrynic acid

Hydrochlorothiazide

Torsemide

Triamterene

Interaction Summary

Concomitant use of gossypol with diuretics, which promote potassium loss, may result in hypokalemia. Triamterene has been found ineffective in preventing this loss.

Discussion

In a study of 120 volunteers from Beijing, administration of gossypol resulted in an average decrease in potassium of 0.062 mEq/L.[1] The loss was not significantly mitigated by potassium administration, with the average potassium loss remaining at 0.056 mEq/L. Volunteers cotreated with triamterene experienced an average potassium loss of 0.11 mEq/L. However, in no patient did the potassium level decrease below 3.0 mEq/L.

In the Chinese district of Nanjing, 7 of 148 men (4.73%) who took gossypol as a contraceptive over a 5-year period developed hypokalemic paralysis.[2] Associated serum potassium levels were

---

Rating Scale:

(1) Significant interaction

(2) Possibly significant interaction

(3) Interaction of relatively little significance

(4) Reported interaction that does not, in fact, exist or is insignificant

2.00 to 2.73 mEq/L. These authors presumed the effect was due to gossypol's inhibitory action on the Na-K ATPase enzyme.

Hence, concomitant use with other agents known to induce potassium loss may result in clinically significant hypokalemia.

Management Suggestions

Patients taking gossypol with diuretics should have their potassium levels monitored at least every 6 weeks for the first 3 months and every 3 months thereafter for the first year.

GLYBURIDE—CHROMIUM

Rating 2

RELATED DRUGS

Acarbose	Miglitol
Acetohexamide	Pioglitazone
Chlorpropamide	Repaglinide
Glimepiride	Rosiglitazone
Glipizide	Tolazamide
Insulin	Tolbutamide
Metformin	Troglitazone

Interaction Summary

Chromium may reduce oral hypoglycemic, or possibly insulin, requirements in patients with diabetes.

Discussion

Some studies, but not all, suggest that chromium supplementation can improve glucose control in patients with diabetes.

A 4-month intervention trial reported in 1997 monitored 180 Chinese men and women with type 2 diabetes, comparing the effects of 1000 µg of chromium, 200 µg of chromium, and placebo.[1] HbA$_{1c}$ values improved significantly after 2 months in

---

Rating Scale:

(1) Significant interaction

(2) Possibly significant interaction

(3) Interaction of relatively little significance

(4) Reported interaction that does not, in fact, exist or is insignificant

the group receiving 1000 μg, and after 4 months in both chromium groups. Fasting glucose was also lower in the higher-dose chromium group at 2 and 4 months, but not in the moderate-dose chromium group. Serum insulin levels decreased significantly in both groups at 2 and 4 months.

A study of 243 patients with type 1 and type 2 diabetes found that chromium supplementation decreased insulin or oral hypoglycemic medication requirements in a significant percentage of cases.[2] However, although this study is commonly reported as a controlled trial, only 10 of the individuals were enrolled in a double-blind protocol. The remainder of the study was open label and, as such, has little validity.

One double-blind study of 30 pregnant women with gestational diabetes found that supplementation with chromium picolinate, 4 or 8 μg/kg, significantly improved blood sugar control as determined by HbA_{1c} measurement, as well as measures of serum glucose and insulin.[3] The lower dose follows standard recommendations for pregnant women; the higher dose did not prove more effective.

On the other hand, chromium supplementation failed to improve glucose tolerance, reduce insulin demand, or alter lipid profiles in 43 outpatients with diabetes.[4]

Although this effect, if real, could be construed as beneficial, it also suggests the potential for inadvertent hypoglycemia among individuals taking hypoglycemic medications.

Management Suggestions

Administering chromium to patients with diabetes may allow a reduction of medication dosage, especially in patients with type 2 diabetes. However, self-administration of chromium could result in hypoglycemia. Question patients closely on this topic, and monitor blood glucose levels carefully if chromium is added.

GLYBURIDE—GINSENG
(PANAX GINSENG, PANAX QUINQUEFOLIUS)

RELATED DRUGS

Acetohexamide

Chlorpropamide

Glipizide

Insulin

Metformin

Tolazamide

Tolbutamide

Troglitazone

OTHER POTENTIALLY IMPLICATED HERBS

Bilberry

Bitter melon (Momordica)

Coccinia indica

Garlic

Gymnema sylvestre

Interaction Summary

Concomitant use may predispose the patient to hypoglycemic responses because ginseng appears to decrease blood glucose levels. Other herbs may possess a similar effect.

Discussion

In an 8-week, double-blind, placebo-controlled study of 36 patients with non-insulin-dependent diabetes, ginseng 200 mg

Rating Scale:

(1) Significant interaction

(2) Possibly significant interaction

(3) Interaction of relatively little significance

(4) Reported interaction that does not, in fact, exist or is insignificant

orally decreased fasting blood glucose compared with placebo
(7.4 ± 1.1 mmol/L and 8.3 ± 1.3 mmol/L, respectively).[1] The
hemoglobin A_{1c} was also lower in patients treated with ginseng
200 mg orally than in those treated with placebo (6% ± 0.3%
and 6.5% ± 1.7%, respectively).[1] The authors attribute these
findings to ginseng-induced increased physical activity in the
treated group, but a cause-and-effect relationship is difficult to
establish.

The effects of American ginseng *(Panax quinquefolius)* have also
been evaluated in two double-blind trials. The first, a double-
blind, placebo-controlled crossover study of nine subjects with
type 2 diabetes, found that a single dose of ginseng 3 g significantly reduced postprandial glycemia.[2] The other study looked
at longer term control of glycemia.[3] In this 8-week trial, American ginseng decreased fasting plasma glucose 9.4% ($P < 0.006$)
versus placebo.

Certain constituents of ginseng have been found to exhibit
hypoglycemic activity, including panaxans A, B, C, E, I, J, K, L,
Q, R, S, T, and U.[4-7] In a study of ginsenoside Rb_2 in streptozotocin-diabetic rats, blood glucose levels were 30% less at day
6 in the ginsenoside Rb_2–treated group versus the controls.[8]
This was accompanied by a 31% decrease in glucose-6-
phosphatase activity in the liver with a significant increase in
glucokinase activity.

Additionally, ginsenosides Rb_1, Rb_2, Rc, and Rg_1 inhibit steroid-
ogenesis induced by a maximally active dose of corticotropin in
isolated rat adrenal cells[9]; hence even in stress conditions, ginseng will most likely continue to exert its hypoglycemic effects.
However, this is confounded by the finding that ginsenoside Rg_1
is also active as a functional ligand of the glucocorticoid receptor.[10] Its potency relative to prednisone is unknown in this regard, but if bound preferentially, it could then decrease the corticosteroid response overall. More study is needed.

Given the apparent ability of ginseng to decrease blood glucose, it is conceivable that it could augment the hypoglycemic response to hypoglycemic agents. Decreased doses may be required or hypoglycemic responses could occur.

However, this has yet to be reported in the clinical literature as a case report, and it has not been formally studied.

Management Suggestions

Patients with diabetes mellitus who elect to use ginseng (or other herbs with hypoglycemic properties) concomitantly with their diabetes medications should be advised to monitor their blood glucose closely. They should be reminded of hypoglycemic indications and be advised to contact a health care provider if these symptoms occur.

GLYBURIDE—VITAMIN E

RELATED DRUGS

Acetohexamide	Insulin
Chlorpropamide	Tolazamide
Glipizide	Tolbutamide

Interaction Summary

High-dose vitamin E might improve glucose transport and thus improve insulin sensitivity. This may mandate a reduction in hypoglycemic drug dosages during concurrent use.

Discussion

In a randomized, double-blind crossover study of glucometabolic effects by Paolisso et al., 15 patients with type 2 diabetes and 10 healthy controls underwent an oral glucose tolerance test or a euglycemic hyperinsulinemic glucose clamp (fixed infusion rate) before and after vitamin E supplementation (DL-alpha-tocopheryl acetate 900 mg/day for 4 months).[1] Before supplementation, the diabetic patients had lower fasting plasma vitamin E concentrations compared to controls. After supplementation, they displayed an increase in plasma vitamin E similar to controls, but a greater reduction in oxygen production (mean ± SEM: 33% ± 4% versus 55% ± 5%; $P < 0.04$), plasma GSSG (oxidized glutathione)/GSH (reduced glutathione) ratio

---

Rating Scale:

(1) Significant interaction

(2) Possibly significant interaction

(3) Interaction of relatively little significance

(4) Reported interaction that does not, in fact, exist or is insignificant

(28% $\pm$ 3% versus 47% $\pm$ 6%; $P < 0.01$), and HBA$_{1c}$ concentrations (5% $\pm$ 2% versus 12% $\pm$ 2%; $P < 0.04$), as well as an increase in total-body glucose disposal (36% $\pm$ 6% versus 19% $\pm$ 2%; $P < 0.03$) and nonoxidative glucose metabolism (57% $\pm$ 7% versus 29% $\pm$ 5%; $P < 0.02$). Significant increases in the GSSG/GSH ratio are believed to contribute to enhanced lipid peroxidation.

Compared to placebo, vitamin E supplementation decreased membrane microviscosity in both diabetic patients and controls, with a stronger effect in the diabetic patients.

In diabetic patients and controls, the percentage increase in plasma vitamin E correlated with the percentage change in oxygen production, GSSG/GSH ratio, membrane microviscosity, total-body glucose disposal, and nonoxidative glucose metabolism.

These findings suggest that high-dose vitamin E supplementation may reduce oxidative stress and improve membrane physical characteristics and related activities in glucose transport, thus enhancing insulin sensitivity.

Another randomized, double-blind crossover study, also conducted by Paolisso et al., found similar results with daily vitamin E supplementation (D-alpha-tocopherol 900 mg/day), which appeared to improve insulin sensitivity in seniors with type 2 diabetes.[2] In the 3-month trial periods, 25 patients took the vitamin or placebo, with a 30-day washout period before crossover. No changes were made in oral hypoglycemic drugs or their dosages. Small but significant reductions in plasma glucose and glycosylated hemoglobin were seen during the treatment phases, without alteration in insulin secretion, suggesting that these benefits were primarily due to enhanced insulin sensitivity. Lipid profiles also improved.

Management Suggestions

Monitor blood glucose levels and adjust the dose of oral hypoglycemic drugs as needed in patients taking vitamin E concurrently.

HALOPERIDOL—KAVA

Rating 2

RELATED DRUGS

Carbidopa	Perphenazine
Chlorpromazine	Pimozide
Eldepryl	Prochlorperazine
Fluphenazine	Promazine
Levodopa	Thioridazine
Loxapine	Thiothixene
Mesoridazine	Trifluoperazine
Metoclopramide	Triflupromazine
Molindone	

Interaction Summary

Preliminary reports suggest that kava may possess dopamine antagonism effects. This may increase the risk of neuroleptic-induced movement disorders, and counter the effect of medications for Parkinson's disease.

Discussion

Four case reports of kava-induced movement disorders suggest that kava may possess central dopamine antagonism activity.

Rating Scale:
(1) Significant interaction
(2) Possibly significant interaction
(3) Interaction of relatively little significance
(4) Reported interaction that does not, in fact, exist or is insignificant

A 28-year-old man experienced an acute attack of involuntary neck extension with forceful upward eye elevation beginning 90 minutes after his first dose of 100 mg kava extract.[1] It resolved spontaneously within 40 minutes. This patient had a history of three episodes of acute dystonic reactions following exposure to promethazine and fluspirilene, all of which were responsive to biperiden.

A 22-year-old woman developed involuntary oral and lingual dyskinesia, tonic head rotation and pain, and twisting trunk movements within 4 hours of taking her first dose of kava extract 100 mg.[1] Her movement disorders resolved following treatment with biperiden.

A third patient, a 63-year-old woman, experienced forceful involuntary oral and lingual dyskinesia after taking kava extract 150 mg three times daily for 4 days.[1] She, too, responded to biperiden.

A fourth patient experienced worsening parkinsonism after ingestion of kava extract 150 mg twice daily for 10 days.[1]

Effects of concomitant use with other dopamine antagonists have not yet been reported. Clearly, more study is needed.

Management Suggestions

Caution should be exercised if kava is used concomitantly with neuroleptics. While this includes well-known antipsychotics such as haloperidol and chlorpromazine, the clinician should remember that dopamine blockers exist in other therapeutic categories (e.g., metoclopramide).

HALOPERIDOL—
PHENYLALANINE

Rating 3

RELATED DRUGS

Acetophenazine	Prochlorperazine
Chlorpromazine	Promazine
Clozapine	Promethazine
Fluphenazine	Propiomazine
Haloperidol	Quetiapine
Loxapine	Risperidone
Mesoridazine	Thiethylperazine
Methotrimeprazine	Thioridazine
Molindone	Thiothixene
Olanzapine	Trifluoperazine
Perphenazine	Triflupromazine
Pimozide	

Interaction Summary

Ingestion of supplemental phenylalanine might worsen symptoms of drug-induced tardive dyskinesia.

Rating Scale:
(1) Significant interaction
(2) Possibly significant interaction
(3) Interaction of relatively little significance
(4) Reported interaction that does not, in fact, exist or is insignificant

Discussion

Tardive dyskinesia (TD), a neurologic disease associated with the use of antipsychotics and other psychotherapeutic agents, is characterized primarily by involuntary movements in the perioral region (tongue, mouth, jaw, eyelids, and face). TD may develop in a substantial percentage of patients taking antipsychotic drugs and no effective treatment has been found. Reports suggest that a reduced ability to clear ingested forms of the large neutral amino acid phenylalanine may be associated with TD. L-Phenylalanine, an essential dietary amino acid, is the starting point of the body's synthesis of the neurotransmitters dopamine, norepinephrine, and epinephrine.

A double-blind, placebo-controlled trial in 18 male schizophrenic patients with TD found that a challenge with phenylalanine 100 mg/kg significantly increased involuntary movements, in contrast to placebo.[1] A statistically significant correlation ($P < 0.05$) between Abnormal Involuntary Movements Scale (AIMS) total scores and plasma phenylalanine levels was found after a loading dose of 100 mg/kg phenylalanine.[2]

Management Suggestions

It might be advisable for patients taking drugs implicated in causing TD, particularly antipsychotic medications, to avoid phenylalanine supplements.

HEPARIN—
PHOSPHATIDYLSERINE

RELATED DRUGS

Anisindione   Warfarin

Dicumarol

Interaction Summary

A combination of phosphatidylserine and phosphatidylethan-olamine enhanced heparin's effect on coagulation time. It is possible that phosphatidylserine alone could produce a similar effect, although such an interaction is presently hypothetical.

Discussion

In an in vitro study, liposomes containing phosphatidylserine (PS) and phosphatidylethanolamine (PE) were found to synergistically stimulate the anticoagulant effect of heparin.[1] Although neither substance produced the same effect alone, it should be recognized that PS is metabolically decarboxylated to PE.[2]

Because many reactions of coagulation proteins occur at phospholipid surfaces, it is possible that high phospholipid concentrations can prolong coagulation time by surface dilution of the bound proteins.

Rating Scale:

(1) Significant interaction

(2) Possibly significant interaction

(3) Interaction of relatively little significance

(4) Reported interaction that does not, in fact, exist or is insignificant

Management Suggestions

Although this interaction is only hypothetical at this time, individuals taking heparin or warfarin should be closely monitored when using this or any other supplement.

HEPARIN—VITAMIN C

Rating 4

Interaction Summary

Weak evidence suggests that very high concentrations of vitamin C reduced the anticoagulant effect of heparin in a test tube.

Discussion

Test tube experiments using dog blood demonstrated that high concentrations of ascorbic acid (vitamin C) can interfere with heparin's anticoagulant effects.[1] It was found that 10 mg of ascorbic acid could neutralize the anticoagulant effects of up to 5 units (about 0.05 mg) of heparin. However, the relevance of this finding to oral use of vitamin C is unclear.

Management Suggestions

The clinical relevance of this interaction is uncertain and no action appears necessary based on this evidence.

Rating Scale:
(1) Significant interaction
(2) Possibly significant interaction

(3) Interaction of relatively little significance
(4) Reported interaction that does not, in fact, exist or is insignificant

IBUPROFEN—FEVERFEW

RELATED DRUGS

Diclofenac	Meclofenamate
Etodolac	Nabumetone
Fenoprofen	Naproxen
Flurbiprofen	Oxaprozin
Indomethacin	Piroxicam
Ketoprofen	Sulindac
Ketorolac	Tolmetin

OTHER POTENTIALLY IMPLICATED HERBS

White willow

Interaction Summary

Feverfew appears to suppress prostaglandin production and might therefore increase NSAID side effects. White willow presents similar risks because it contains salicylates.

Discussion

Feverfew extract (50 or 150 μl/ml) has been shown to suppress 86% to 88% of prostaglandin production without an effect on cyclooxygenase.[1] Furthermore, lactones (parthenolide and epoxy-artemorin) isolated from feverfew have been found to be

---

Rating Scale:
(1) Significant interaction
(2) Possibly significant interaction
(3) Interaction of relatively little significance
(4) Reported interaction that does not, in fact, exist or is insignificant

inhibitory with IC_{50} values ranging from approximately 1 to 5 μg/ml, irreversibly inhibiting eicosanoid generation.[2] Tanetin, a lipophilic avonol (6-hydroxykaempferol 3,7,4'-trimethyl ether) has also been identified as a feverfew constituent that inhibits generation of proinflammatory eicosanoids.[3]

These findings suggest that concomitant use of feverfew and NSAIDs might increase risk of gastropathy and nephropathy.

Management Suggestions

It would appear to be in the best interest of the patient not to combine feverfew and NSAIDs.

INDINAVIR—ST. JOHN'S WORT

NOTE: See Table I in Guengerich, 1999, for the most comprehensive list of CYP3A4 and *p*-glycoprotein drug substrates.[1]

RELATED DRUGS

Cyclosporine

CYP3A4 and P-glycoprotein
drug substrates, including
cyclosporine, digoxin, oral
contraceptives, warfarin,
theophylline, simvastatin,
lovastatin, and atorvastatin
(but not pravastatin)

HIV protease inhibitors

Interaction Summary

Concomitant use of St. John's wort extract causes increased metabolism of the HIV protease inhibitor indinavir to a sufficient extent that antiretroviral resistance and outright treatment failure are real possibilities. A similar effect is likely to occur with other protease inhibitors. In February 2000, the U.S. FDA issued a warning to health care providers regarding this risk.

Discussion

A commentary by Ernst raised attention to several reports implicating induction of CYP3A4 by St. John's wort.[2] Because

---

Rating Scale:
(1) Significant interaction
(2) Possibly significant
    interaction

(3) Interaction of relatively little
    significance
(4) Reported interaction that
    does not, in fact, exist or is
    insignificant

many HIV protease inhibitors are known substrates for CYP3A4, investigators at the National Institute of Allergy and Infectious Diseases performed an open-label study in eight healthy volunteers (6 male, 2 female, ages 29 to 50 years) to investigate the effect of St. John's wort on the pharmacokinetics of the most widely used HIV protease inhibitor, indinavir.[3] Patients served as their own controls, first receiving four 800-mg oral doses of indinavir at 8-hour intervals, with plasma drug levels determined at 0.5 to 8 hours following the final dose. All patients then received three doses per day of a standardized (0.3% hypericin) St. John's wort product for 14 days and were then subjected to the same indinavir dosing and monitoring paradigm described earlier.

The area under the curve for the 8-hour indinavir dosing interval (AUC_{0-8}) decreased by a mean of 57% after St. John's wort dosing (30.8 ± 8.4 to 12.3 ± 4.7). The 8-hour indinavir concentration (C_8) was reduced 49% to 99% in all patients, from a mean of 0.493 μg/ml with indinavir alone to 0.048 μg/ml after St. John's wort.

Although these studies were done in healthy volunteers, the authors concluded that the large decrease in indinavir concentrations after St. John's wort might cause antiretroviral resistance and treatment failure if similar responses occurred in HIV-infected individuals.

Increasing evidence suggests that St. John's wort induces CYP3A and intestinal p-glycoprotein.[8,9] For example, one trial found that St. John's wort decreased plasma concentrations of simvastatin but not pravastatin.[10] Simvastatin is metabolized by CYP3A4 in the gut and liver, while pravastatin is primarily metabolized through non-CYP pathways.

It should be noted that there exists one high-quality, but small, prospective study[4] suggesting that St. John's wort is *without* significant effect on CYP3A4 or another major cytochrome P450, CYP2D6. The discrepancy between this and other reports may be due to the variable quality of St. John's wort preparations used in each study. In addition, another report using urinary

6-beta-hydroxycortisol/cortisol ratios as a measure of CYP3A4 activity in human volunteers before and after 14 days of St. John's wort revealed large interindividual variations in CYP3A4 induction among subjects (mean 114% ± 95% change from baseline, range of −25% to 259%).[5]

Although hypericin is the most likely St. John's wort component mediating CYP1A2 induction,[6] the compound responsible for CYP3A4 induction appears to be hyperforin, one of the active ingredients in the herb. Of 15 St. John's wort components tested, hyperforin was the only one shown to induce CYP3A4 in human hepatocytes.[7] This effect appears to be mediated by hyperforin binding to and activating the hepatic transcription factor, PXR. In fact, hyperforin is at least 50-fold more potent in binding PXR than rifampicin, the classic CYP3A4 inducer. This report raises another issue: the known chemical instability of hyperforin may partly account for the variable CYP3A4 induction observed with different St. John's wort preparations.

Management Suggestions

The possibility of patients with HIV taking St. John's wort must be taken seriously. Patients infected with HIV or any other chronic illness are predisposed to depression and may choose to self-medicate with St. John's wort in the false belief that, because it is "natural," it is safe. In addition, older literature suggests that St. John's wort might have anti-HIV effects (although controlled trials have not proven promising). St. John's wort may also reduce serum levels of nevirapine.[11] The result may be treatment failure.

In addition, if drug levels are optimized in an individual already using St. John's wort, abrupt discontinuation of the herb could result in rebound toxicity. For these reasons, physician vigilance is warranted. Direct questioning and counseling are advised, because patients may not volunteer information regarding their use of herbs.

INSULIN—VANADIUM

Rating 3

RELATED DRUGS

Acetohexamide	Pioglitazone
Chlorpropamide	Repaglinide
Glimepiride	Rosiglitazone
Glipizide	Tolazamide
Glyburide	Tolbutamide
Metformin	Troglitazone

Interaction Summary

Vanadium may reduce insulin requirements in patients with diabetes.

Discussion

Vanadium is known to be an essential trace element in animals, but its essentiality in humans is not established. It appears to have insulin-like effects in vitro, and antidiabetic efficacy in animal models.[1] In clinical studies in humans, vanadium produced no consistent effects on glucose control in patients with type 1 diabetes, but requirements of daily insulin fell by 14%. In patients with type 2 diabetes, however, vanadium treatment increased insulin sensitivity, resulting in less glycogenolysis and improved glycogen storage. As with the animal studies, most of these metabolic effects were sustained for up to 2 weeks following treatment.

Vanadyl sulfate was used in a single-blind, placebo-controlled trial involving seven patients with type 2 diabetes and six non-diabetic individuals.[2] At 100 mg/day, the compound improved hepatic and skeletal muscle insulin sensitivity in the moderately obese subjects with diabetes, in part by enhancing insulin's inhibitory effect on lipolysis. This effect was not seen in the non-diabetic subjects. It has been hypothesized that vanadyl sulfate may improve a defect in insulin signaling that is specific to type 2 diabetes.

Animal studies suggest that vanadium in high doses can lead to accumulation and toxicity.[3,4]

Management Suggestions

Monitor blood glucose levels carefully and adjust the dose of insulin or oral hypoglycemic drug as needed in patients taking this combination. Advise patients to report indications of hypoglycemia.

IRON—CALCIUM CARBONATE

Rating 3

RELATED DRUGS

Calcium acetate

Calcium carbonate

Calcium citrate

Calcium glubionate

Calcium gluconate

Calcium lactate

Calcium phosphate

Tricalcium phosphate

RELATED SUPPLEMENTS

Ferrous fumarate

Ferrous gluconate

Ferrous sulfate

Iron polysaccharide

Interaction Summary

Calcium-containing antacids and other calcium supplements may reduce iron absorption.

Discussion

The cumulative findings suggest that calcium reduces iron absorption primarily by competing with it for final transport from intestinal cells into the blood circulation.

A single-blind, placebo-controlled crossover study of 13 healthy postmenopausal women found that both supplemental calcium carbonate and hydroxyapatite (a calcium phosphate compound)

Rating Scale:

(1) Significant interaction

(2) Possibly significant interaction

(3) Interaction of relatively little significance

(4) Reported interaction that does not, in fact, exist or is insignificant

given concurrently with a meal reduced iron absorption from the meal by over 40%.[1] Iron in the meal was present as the non-heme form (from plant-derived foods).

A calcium chloride supplement at doses of 300 to 600 mg taken with meals was found to reduce iron absorption from meals by 50% to 60% in healthy volunteers.[2] Even dietary calcium (as milk or cheese) in the amount of 165 mg reduced dietary iron absorption by the same 50% to 60%. The absorption of heme iron (the most absorbable form, present in meats) was also significantly reduced.

Similarly, another study involving 61 volunteers found that regular use of calcium supplements with meals may make it more difficult to meet daily iron requirements.[3]

Taking a calcium supplement (calcium carbonate, citrate, or phosphate) and an iron supplement (ferrous sulfate) with food significantly reduced absorption of the iron supplement. Furthermore, calcium supplements reduced absorption of nonheme iron present in the meal. Interestingly, while calcium carbonate supplements had no effect on absorption of the iron supplement when taken between meals, the other two calcium supplements did reduce the iron supplement's absorption.

A randomized, placebo-controlled study of 109 free-living post-menopausal women appears to contradict these other studies, but close examination suggests a possible explanation.[4] Researchers found that 1000 mg of calcium carbonate taken daily with meals did not reduce the body's iron stores. However, these women also had a relatively high daily dietary intake (215 mg) of vitamin C, which is known to enhance iron absorption.

Management Suggestions

Antacids containing calcium, as well as calcium supplements, should be administered apart from meals. However, if any form of calcium other than calcium carbonate is used, it may be advisable to monitor body iron stores periodically.

IRON—H_2 ANTAGONISTS

RELATED DRUGS

Cimetidine

Famotidine

Lansoprazole

Nizatidine

Omeprazole

Rabeprazole sodium

Ranitidine

OTHER POTENTIALLY IMPLICATED SUPPLEMENTS

Ferrous fumarate

Ferrous gluconate

Ferrous sulfate

Iron polysaccharide

Minerals, Zinc

Interaction Summary

By increasing gastric pH levels, H_2 antagonists and other drugs that inhibit gastric acid secretion might interfere with the absorption of iron and zinc and possibly other minerals that are absorbed best under acidic conditions.

Discussion

The pH of the stomach is one of many factors affecting iron and zinc absorption. It is well known that gastric acid secretion affects iron absorption. High levels of acidity separate ferric ions from proteins with a molecular weight larger than 10,000.[1]

Rating Scale:
(1) Significant interaction
(2) Possibly significant interaction
(3) Interaction of relatively little significance
(4) Reported interaction that does not, in fact, exist or is insignificant

Conversely, a reduction in acidity allows for formation of insoluble complexes in the stomach.

Zinc absorption appears to be affected similarly. A study with 11 volunteers compared the rate of absorption of zinc in individuals given either H₂ blockers or no treatment.[2] Gastric acidity was monitored via nasogastric tube. Researchers found that cimetidine and ranitidine significantly reduced serum zinc levels.

Other minerals absorbed best under acidic conditions might be similarly affected by agents that increase stomach pH.

Management Suggestions

Multimineral supplementation may be advisable in patients taking H₂ antagonists or proton pump inhibitors to help ensure nutriture of iron, zinc, and other minerals. However, iron supplementation is not recommended in the absence of demonstrated iron deficiency. On the other hand, marginal zinc deficiency is common,[3-7] and supplementation with recommended nutritional dosages of zinc may be warranted.

IRON SALTS—BEVERAGE TEAS

OTHER POTENTIALLY IMPLICATED HERBS

Agrimony
Apricot
Artichoke
Avens
Bilberry
Birch leaf
Blackberry leaf
Black tea
Blackthorn berry
Blue flag
Boldo
Borage
Burnet
Calamus
Cascara
Cassia
Chamomile
Clivers
Cohosh (black)
Cola
Coltsfoot leaf
Comfrey

Cornsilk
Cowslip
Damiana
Drosera
Elder
Eucalyptus leaf
Eyebright
Feverfew
Frangula
Gentian
Ground ivy
Hawthorn
Hempnettle
Holythistle
Hops
Horehound
Horse chestnut
Ispaghula
Jambolan bark
Juniper berry
Knotweed
Lady's mantle

Rating Scale:
(1) Significant interaction
(2) Possibly significant interaction
(3) Interaction of relatively little significance
(4) Reported interaction that does not, in fact, exist or is insignificant

OTHER POTENTIALLY IMPLICATED HERBS—cont'd

Lady's slipper	Rose flower
Lavender flower	Sage leaf
Lemon balm	Sassafras
Lime flower	Saw palmetto
Linden flower	Skullcap
Marshmallow	Slippery elm
Meadowsweet	Squill
Mistletoe	Stone root
Motherwort	Tansy
Nettle	Thyme
Oak bark	Uva ursi
Peppermint leaf	Valerian
Pilewort	Vervain
Plantain	Walnut leaf
Poplar	White dead nettle flower
Potentilla	Willow
Prickly ash	Witch hazel leaf and bark
Queen's delight	Woody nightshade stem
Raspberry	Wormwood
Rhatany root	Yarrow
Rhubarb	Yellow dock

Interaction Summary

If tea is ingested concomitantly with iron supplements, there is a concern that iron absorption may be diminished.

Discussion

Tannins (also referred to as *tannic acid*) are water-soluble polyphenols found in many types of beverage teas.[1,2] Evidence suggests that they may decrease the absorption of various nutrients.[3] Chief among these is iron. In a study of 122 healthy infants from the age of 6 to 12 months, the ingestion of herbal teas (median intake: 250 ml) was associated with a significantly higher incidence of microcytic anemia (32.6% versus 3.5% in non-tea drinkers).[4] Herbal teas with tannin contents from less than 10 mg tannic acid/g dry herb up to 117 mg tannic acid/g dry herb have been found to inhibit iron absorption if the herbal tea is consumed concurrently.[5] Hence, it is of concern that if a patient is ingesting over-the-counter ferrous sulfate, gluconate, or one of the other salts for treatment of microcytic anemia, concomitant ingestion of tea may inhibit adequate absorption of iron. No intervention studies have addressed this possible drug-herb interaction, but sufficient data exist as noted above to raise concern.

Management Suggestions

Patients prescribed ferrous sulfate, gluconate, or other salts should be advised not to ingest these tablets concomitantly with beverage teas until this potential drug-herb interaction has been adequately investigated.

ISOTRETINOIN—VITAMIN A

Interaction Summary

Isotretinoin may have additive toxic effects if combined with retinol (vitamin A).

Discussion

Vitamin A in high doses (e.g., above 50,000 IU daily) can lead to accumulation and toxicity. Because isotretinoin is an isomer of all-*trans* retinoic acid, which is a metabolite of retinol (vitamin A), this combination could produce additive toxicity.

Management Suggestions

The combination of vitamin A and isotretinoin should be avoided.

Rating Scale:
(1) Significant interaction
(2) Possibly significant interaction

(3) Interaction of relatively little significance
(4) Reported interaction that does not, in fact, exist or is insignificant

LEVODOPA/CARBIDOPA—BCAAs

OTHER POTENTIALLY IMPLICATED SUPPLEMENTS
Amino acid supplements

Interaction Summary

Like dietary protein, BCAAs (branched-chain amino acids) and other amino acid supplements may temporarily decrease the effectiveness of levodopa.

Discussion

BCAAs and other amino acid supplements may have effects similar to meals high in protein. High-protein meals can interfere strikingly with levodopa therapy and aggravate the symptoms of Parkinson's disease.[1] After dietary protein is broken down into amino acids in the gastrointestinal tract, the absorption process is facilitated by amino acid transport mechanisms. Because levodopa is a derivative of the amino acid phenylalanine, competition between the drug levodopa and dietary amino acids may occur. There may also be competition for the carrier that transports amino acids into the brain.

Management Suggestions

It may be advisable to avoid BCAAs and other amino acid supplements during levodopa therapy for Parkinson's disease.

Rating Scale:
(1) Significant interaction
(2) Possibly significant interaction
(3) Interaction of relatively little significance
(4) Reported interaction that does not, in fact, exist or is insignificant

LEVODOPA/CARBIDOPA—IRON

Rating 1

RELATED SUPPLEMENTS

Ferrous fumarate

Ferrous gluconate

Ferrous sulfate

Iron polysaccharide

Interaction Summary

Iron decreases the effect of levodopa in Parkinson's disease by interfering with the absorption of both levodopa and carbidopa.

Discussion

Both levodopa and carbidopa accelerate the oxidation of ferrous iron to ferric iron. Ferric iron binds levodopa strongly in a 3:1 levodopa/iron complex and so would be expected to substantially reduce levodopa's bioavailability.[1] Ferrous sulfate has been found to decrease levodopa AUC by 51% and peak levels by 55% in healthy subjects. In patients taking levodopa and carbidopa, ferrous sulfate reduced levodopa AUC by 30% and peak levels by 47%, and reduced carbidopa AUC by 75%, with clinical deterioration of Parkinson's disease.

Management Suggestions

Administer iron supplements and levodopa formulations as far apart as is feasible. Increase the dosage of levodopa/carbidopa based on clinical response.

Rating Scale:

(1) Significant interaction

(2) Possibly significant interaction

(3) Interaction of relatively little significance

(4) Reported interaction that does not, in fact, exist or is insignificant

LITHIUM—HERBAL DIURETICS

Rating 2

OTHER POTENTIALLY IMPLICATED HERBS

Broom
Buchu
Burdock
Cornsilk
Celery seed
Cleavers
Couchgrass
Dandelion
Elder broom

Goldenrod
Gravel root
Horsetail
Juniper
Nettle
Parsely
Uva ursi
Wild carrot

Interaction Summary

Numerous herbs are suspected or known to have diuretic properties, including broom, buchu, burdock, cornsilk, celery seed, cleavers, couchgrass, dandelion, elder, goldenrod, gravel root, horsetail, juniper, nettle, parsley, uva ursi, and wild carrot. Individuals on lithium therapy who use diuretic herbs may experience dehydration and resulting lithium toxicity.

Discussion

A 26-year-old woman had been stabilized on 900 mg bid of lithium for 5 months.[1] She presented to the emergency room

Rating Scale:
(1) Significant interaction
(2) Possibly significant interaction
(3) Interaction of relatively little significance
(4) Reported interaction that does not, in fact, exist or is insignificant

complaining of grogginess and exhibited coarse tremor, unsteady gait, and nystagmus. Her lithium level was 5.5 mmol/L. Questioning revealed that she had a 2-week history of using an herbal preparation for weight loss. The combination included a number of herbs believed to exert diuretic effects, including buchu, corn silk, horsetail, juniper, parsley, and uva ursi. It appears likely that these herbs were responsible for the development of lithium toxicity.

Management Suggestions

Individuals on lithium therapy should be cautioned against using herbs with diuretic properties. Such herbs are frequently included in products advertised as promoting weight loss. Individuals who insist on using such herbs should be advised of the symptoms of lithium toxicity and should undergo frequent lithium level measurements.

MAGNESIUM—FUROSEMIDE

RELATED DRUGS

Bendroflumethiazide
Benzthiazide
Bumetanide
Chlorothiazide
Chlorthalidone
Ethacrynic acid
Hydrochlorothiazide
Hydroflumethiazide

Indapamide
Methyclothiazide
Metolazone
Polythiazide
Quinethazone
Torsemide
Trichlormethiazide

Interaction Summary

Like thiazide diuretics, loop diuretics such as furosemide increase the urinary excretion of magnesium along with sodium and potassium. In some cases, this may lead to a magnesium deficiency.

Discussion

Loop and thiazide diuretics increase the urinary excretion of magnesium along with sodium and potassium.[1,2] The extent of magnesium depletion may depend on the type of diuretic, dose, and duration of therapy.[3]

Rating Scale:
(1) Significant interaction
(2) Possibly significant interaction

(3) Interaction of relatively little significance
(4) Reported interaction that does not, in fact, exist or is insignificant

If magnesium depletion is prolonged, the body may appropriate the mineral from bones to maintain blood magnesium levels. This is one reason that serum magnesium levels can be normal in the presence of tissue depletion and that low serum levels may indicate a significant magnesium deficiency.[1,4]

Nonetheless, in most cases, measuring serum magnesium concentration and urinary magnesium excretion is sufficient to diagnose magnesium deficiency.[1] Occasionally, the parenteral magnesium load test may be required to assess magnesium status.

Refractory hypokalemia can be caused by hypomagnesemia and can be corrected by magnesium supplementation.[5]

Normal magnesium (and potassium) status in patients on long-term diuretic therapy may be restored by giving oral magnesium, but supplementation needs to be maintained for 6 months.[3] Magnesium gluconate tends to cause less diarrhea than other forms and so is better tolerated.[1] Another option is to add a magnesium-potassium–sparing diuretic.[3] For example, 5 to 10 mg of amiloride may negate the magnesium-wasting effect of 40 mg of furosemide.[1] However, hypomagnesemia was also found in 12% of patients taking a combination of furosemide and amiloride.[3] Severe or symptomatic magnesium deficiency is usually treated with magnesium sulfate given IV or IM.[1]

Management Suggestions

Oral magnesium supplementation may be advisable for patients on long-term diuretic therapy. An alternative is to add a magnesium-potassium–sparing diuretic.

MAGNESIUM—
ORAL CONTRACEPTIVES

RELATED DRUGS

Ethinyl estradiol

Estradiol

Estrogen

Estropipate

Interaction Summary

Oral contraceptives (OCs) or estrogen replacement therapy may deplete body stores of magnesium by increasing its uptake and utilization by soft tissues and bone.

Discussion

Estrogen enhances magnesium utilization by moving the mineral from the blood into body tissues and bone.[1] A 1991 study in 32 women found a 26% decrease in serum magnesium after 6 months of OC use (ethinyl estradiol 0.03 mg and levonorgestrel 0.15 mg) compared to baseline levels, which were normal in all the women.[2] Serum magnesium levels decreased from 0.82 to 0.61 mmol/L ($P < 0.001$). Similar findings have been observed during pregnancy and during estrogen replacement therapy in menopause. Though no clinical findings associated with the decreased magnesium levels were noted in this study, signs of symptomatic hypomagnesemia include appetite loss, nausea and

---

Rating Scale:

(1) Significant interaction

(2) Possibly significant interaction

(3) Interaction of relatively little significance

(4) Reported interaction that does not, in fact, exist or is insignificant

vomiting, sleepiness, weakness, muscle spasms, tremors, and personality changes.

Management Suggestions

Consider magnesium supplementation for patients taking OCs or estrogen replacement therapy who have suboptimal magnesium intake or compromised serum magnesium levels.

MAGNESIUM—POTASSIUM-SPARING DIURETICS

Rating 3

RELATED DRUGS

Amiloride   Triamterene

Spironolactone

Interaction Summary

Potassium-sparing diuretics may reduce urinary magnesium excretion.

Discussion

According to animal studies, potassium-sparing diuretics may reduce urinary excretion of magnesium as well as potassium.[1] In some cases, this effect may be useful. For instance, thiazide diuretics and loop diuretics increase the urinary excretion of magnesium along with sodium and potassium,[2] and adding a potassium-sparing diuretic may help counter this magnesium loss.[3] However, combined magnesium supplementation and treatment with potassium-sparing diuretics could conceivably create a risk of hypermagnesemia.

Management Suggestions

Individuals taking potassium-sparing diuretics should use magnesium supplements with caution.

Rating Scale:

(1) Significant interaction

(2) Possibly significant interaction

(3) Interaction of relatively little significance

(4) Reported interaction that does not, in fact, exist or is insignificant

MANGANESE—CALCIUM CARBONATE

Rating 3

Interaction Summary

Though findings of numerous studies have conflicted, in some cases it appears that calcium-containing antacids may reduce the absorption of manganese. The clinical significance of this finding, however, is not clear.

Discussion

Calcium-containing antacids may interfere with manganese absorption. Manganese ions bind at the same intracellular sites as calcium ions, and it is possible that these two minerals may compete for a variety of solubilizing or chelating agents.[1]

In one study, six adult subjects were administered a series of manganese tolerance tests to determine the influence of various minerals on plasma manganese uptake.[1] Subjects took 40 mg of supplemental manganese chloride alone or with either supplemental calcium carbonate (800 mg) or milk (an amount containing 800 mg of calcium). Both calcium sources greatly reduced the plasma uptake of manganese.

Another study of 60 healthy adults used a radionuclide technique to measure manganese absorption. Manganese was added to various test meals (human milk, infant formula, and wheat

Rating Scale:
(1) Significant interaction
(2) Possibly significant interaction

(3) Interaction of relatively little significance
(4) Reported interaction that does not, in fact, exist or is insignificant

bread) along with other dietary factors, including phytate, phosphate, ascorbic acid, iron, and magnesium. Only the addition of calcium to human milk in amounts corresponding to that present in cow's milk resulted in a significant decrease in manganese absorption.[2]

Management Suggestions

To avoid a potential absorptive interaction, administer calcium-containing antacids 2 to 3 hours apart from manganese supplements and from meals.

METHYLDOPA—IRON

RELATED SUPPLEMENTS

Ferrous fumarate	Ferrous sulfate
Ferrous gluconate	Iron polysaccharide

Interaction Summary

Ferrous sulfate and ferrous gluconate can substantially decrease the absorption of methyldopa and interfere with blood pressure control.

Discussion

In a randomized crossover trial enrolling 12 subjects, absorption of methyldopa, 500 mg, was reduced by 73% with ferrous sulfate, 325 mg, and by 61% with ferrous gluconate, 600 mg.[1] To determine the clinical consequences of the interaction with ferrous sulfate, five subjects on chronic methyldopa therapy for hypertension were given ferrous sulfate for 2 weeks. Both systolic and diastolic blood pressure increased in four patients. These increases in blood pressure were substantial in three of the patients. Blood pressure decreased in all patients after the iron supplement was stopped.

Rating Scale:
(1) Significant interaction
(2) Possibly significant interaction

(3) Interaction of relatively little significance
(4) Reported interaction that does not, in fact, exist or is insignificant

In a trial involving four subjects, ferrous sulfate caused a 42% decrease in methyldopa absorption even when given 2 hours before the drug.[2]

Possible mechanisms for the decreased absorption of methyldopa include chelation of methyldopa by iron as well as alterations in the gastrointestinal transit time of methyldopa past its site of absorption in the proximal small intestine.[1]

Management Suggestions

Because iron may significantly reduce methyldopa absorption even when taken 2 hours before the drug, it would be advisable to separate administration times by as long as possible.

NEFAZODONE—
ST. JOHN'S WORT

Rating 2

RELATED DRUGS

Selective serotonin
reuptake inhibitor
(SSRI) antidepressants

Tramadol

Trazodone

OTHER POTENTIALLY IMPLICATED HERBS

Ayahuasca

Interaction Summary

Concomitant use of St. John's wort extract may cause peripheral serotonin overload (serotonin syndrome), especially problematic in elderly patients. The herb ayahuasca, which possesses alkaloids with MAO inhibitor action, may present a similar risk.

Discussion

St. John's wort may act similarly to SSRIs. In one study, researchers observed that St. John's wort extract caused down-regulation of serotonin receptors in cultured rat neuroblastoma cells.[1] Subchronic treatment in rodents has shown up-regulation of 5-HT2 receptors in the frontal cortex.[2] Another study noted a 50% inhibition of synaptosomal uptake of serotonin, dopamine, and norepinephrine in mouse brain preparations at

---

Rating Scale:

(1) Significant interaction

(2) Possibly significant
    interaction

(3) Interaction of relatively little
    significance

(4) Reported interaction that
    does not, in fact, exist or is
    insignificant

realistic concentrations of standard St. John's wort extracts.[3] This effect was found to correlate closely with hyperforin concentration in the herbal preparation.[4]

Based on these findings, concerns have arisen regarding the possible development of serotonin syndrome if St. John's wort is combined with SSRIs or other pharmaceuticals that can increase serotonin levels.

Seven case reports (four with nefazodone and one each with sertraline, trazadone, and paroxetine) have been published regarding patients concomitantly taking St. John's wort who experienced symptoms of "serotonin syndrome."[5-8] This peripheral overload of serotonin, caused by inhibition of reuptake primarily of platelet stores of serotonin, can cause restlessness, myalgia, muscle rigidity, mental confusion, tremor, nausea, and gastrointestinal upset.

Serotonin syndrome can progress to acute delirium and has proven fatal.[9] Hence this possible drug-herb interaction needs to be taken very seriously.

The herb ayahuasca, a psychoactive beverage from the Amazon, contains harmala alkaloids with MAO inhibitor properties. One case report suggests that the combination of fluoxetine and ayahuasca caused the development of serotonin syndrome.[10]

Management Suggestions

In general, concomitant use of more than one SSRI should be avoided in all patients with the exception of patients refractory to one agent who are being switched to another. In this regard, St. John's wort should be considered equivalent to SSRI pharmaceuticals. If combined, the patient should be closely monitored for central nervous system depression, headache, sweating, and/or agitation. Keep in mind the long half-life of some SSRIs, especially fluoxetine. The half-life of hyperforin (the leading candidate for active ingredient in St. John's wort) is thought to be about 9 hours.[11]

NIACIN—ISONIAZID

Rating 3

OTHER POTENTIALLY IMPLICATED SUPPLEMENTS

Niacinamide   Vitamin B_3

Nicotinamide

Interaction Summary

As a vitamin B_6–antagonist, isoniazid can interfere with the biosynthesis of niacin, which requires vitamin B_6. In some cases, this may lead to the development of the niacin-deficiency disease pellagra.

Discussion

A study in rats indicated that the antituberculosis drug isoniazid does not cause niacin deficiency by directly interfering with the conversion of tryptophan to niacin.[1] Instead, it appears that isoniazid's well-known interference with vitamin B_6—which is necessary for the metabolism of tryptophan to niacin—is the primary mechanism.

A patient developed signs and symptoms suggestive of pellagra after 10 months of isoniazid therapy (with vitamin B_6).[2] Her pellagra-like illness responded rapidly to withdrawal of isoniazid and administration of nicotinic acid. Vitamin B_6 and niacin

---

Rating Scale:

(1) Significant interaction

(2) Possibly significant interaction

(3) Interaction of relatively little significance

(4) Reported interaction that does not, in fact, exist or is insignificant

(200 mg daily) were continued for another month and stopped. In 2 weeks, the prior skin eruption and diarrhea reappeared. The symptoms quickly cleared up after the B vitamins were restarted, and vitamin therapy was continued for several more months and stopped with no further problems.

A retrospective study found eight undiagnosed cases of pellagra among 106 patients with tuberculosis who had been treated with isoniazid.[3] Four of the eight patients had no skin lesions, but neuropathologically they showed severe chromatolytic neurons in the same distribution as in the other four cases, as well as psychosis and other symptoms suggestive of pellagra. All eight patients had been hospitalized and may not have had much sun exposure. Because pellagrous dermatitis is a photosensitive lesion and appears on exposed parts of the body, some bedridden patients may not develop typical skin lesions; it is believed that these patients had *pellagra sine pelle agra*, or pellagra psychosis without skin lesions. For this reason, pellagra should be suspected whenever tuberculosis patients treated with isoniazid develop mental, neurologic, or gastrointestinal symptoms, even in the absence of the typical pellagra-associated dermatitis.

Management Suggestions

Niacin administration should be considered during isoniazid therapy to prevent drug-induced pellagra, particularly in poorly nourished patients. The most effective niacin dosage has not been determined, but 200 mg daily was used in one study.

NIFEDIPINE—PEPPERMINT OIL

Rating 2

RELATED DRUGS

Amlodipine	Nicardipine
Bepridil	Nimodipine
Diltiazem	Nisoldipine
Felodipine	Nitrendipine
Isradipine	Verapamil

Interaction Summary

Peppermint oil may alter the effectiveness of nifedipine.

Discussion

Peppermint oil has been advocated for the treatment of irritable bowel syndrome due to its antispasmodic action on isolated segments of ileum in animal models (i.e., cats and rabbits).[1] This potential benefit may be related to peppermint oil's calcium channel–blocking activity.[2]

When tested on guinea pig ileum suspended in modified Tyrode's solution, peppermint oil was found to inhibit carbachol-induced influx of extracellular calcium.[3] Whether peppermint oil can potentiate the effects of calcium channel blockers, or, through competition for binding sites, decrease their effectiveness, remains unclear.

Rating Scale:
(1) Significant interaction
(2) Possibly significant interaction
(3) Interaction of relatively little significance
(4) Reported interaction that does not, in fact, exist or is insignificant

Management Suggestions

Scant information suggests peppermint oil may act competitively with nifedipine. Although it is conceivable that nifedipine's effectiveness may be diminished, this has not yet been observed clinically. In contrast, theoretically, the effects could be additive or synergistic. Based on this minimal information, close monitoring is advised if both agents are used together.

NITROFURANTOIN—
MAGNESIUM

Rating 3

Interaction Summary

Magnesium supplements may interfere with absorption of nitrofurantoin.

Discussion

Coadministering nitrofurantoin with magnesium trisilicate to healthy subjects reduced the drug's excretion, presumably reflecting a decrease in its absorption.[1] In 10 volunteers given nitrofurantoin 100 mg with a magnesium-aluminum antacid, the bioavailability of nitrofurantoin was reduced by about 25%.[2] However, no studies have yet evaluated whether this effect is clinically significant.

Management Suggestions

If the combination of magnesium and nitrofurantoin can't be avoided, it would be advisable to separate administration times by as long as possible.

Rating Scale:
(1) Significant interaction
(2) Possibly significant interaction

(3) Interaction of relatively little significance
(4) Reported interaction that does not, in fact, exist or is insignificant

NITROGLYCERIN—
N-ACETYL CYSTEINE

Rating 3

RELATED DRUGS

Isosorbide dinitrate   Isosorbide mononitrate

Interaction Summary

N-acetyl cysteine (NAC) has been tried as a treatment to reverse the tolerance that develops to the vascular and antianginal effects of nitrates. However, this combination appears to increase the incidence of nitrate side effects, including severe headache.

Discussion

A major problem with preventive nitrate therapy is the development of tolerance to the vascular and antianginal effects of these drugs when they are given continuously. The cause of nitrate tolerance is not completely understood and may involve numerous factors. One premise is that continuous nitrate administration leads to depletion of the reduced sulfhydryl groups that are necessary for nitrate-induced vasodilation.[1] *N*-acetyl cysteine, a donor of sulfhydryl groups, has been tried as a way to neutralize the tolerance to nitrate therapy. However, side effects, most notably headache, also increase.

Rating Scale:
(1) Significant interaction
(2) Possibly significant interaction

(3) Interaction of relatively little significance
(4) Reported interaction that does not, in fact, exist or is insignificant

In a double-blind, placebo-controlled trial of 200 individuals with unstable angina who were followed for 4 months, the addition of nitroglycerin (transdermal patch) and NAC to conventional therapy (e.g., aspirin, beta-blockers, calcium channel blockers) reduced adverse outcomes—death, myocardial infarction, or refractory angina requiring revascularization.[1] Adverse events occurred in 31% of patients receiving nitroglycerin, 42% of those receiving NAC, and 13% of those receiving the combination of nitroglycerin and NAC, compared to 39% for placebo ($P = 0.0052$). However, the nitroglycerin-NAC combination therapy increased the incidence of intolerable headache, which was almost twice as frequent as in patients receiving nitroglycerin alone. Similar exacerbation of headache has been seen in other trials.[2]

Several studies have suggested a beneficial effect of NAC on nitrate tolerance. One study of 19 subjects—17 with coronary artery disease and 2 without it—found that the coronary vasodilating effect of intracoronary nitroglycerin injections was decreased by 24-hour IV nitroglycerin infusion, indicating the development of partial tolerance, which was reversed by IV infusion of NAC.[3] A study of 20 patients with coronary artery disease found that susceptibility to nitrate tolerance was higher in venous than arterial circulation, and that NAC was effective in reversing nitroglycerin tolerance in venous circulation.[4] In a study involving 11 participants, nitroglycerin (0.06 µg/kg/min) was infused for 20 minutes immediately after and 2 hours after pretreatment with NAC (100 mg/kg) or placebo.[2] NAC was found to significantly potentiate and prolong nitroglycerin-induced dilation of the temporal artery only after the first nitroglycerin infusion, indicating that the effect of NAC was short lasting.

However, not all studies have found NAC to be effective. A small double-blind, placebo-controlled study found that chronic oral administration of NAC failed to prevent the development of tolerance to the antianginal or hemodynamic effects of glyceryl trinitrate.[5] An earlier study by the same authors found similarly negative results.[6]

Management Suggestions

The use of *N*-acetyl cysteine may in some cases prevent the development of nitrate tolerance. However, chronic use of NAC in patients taking nitrates may cause side effects that limit its clinical use.

NSAIDs—GOSSYPOL

RELATED DRUGS

Aspirin	Meclofenamate
Diclofenac	Nabumetone
Etodolac	Naproxen
Fenoprofen	Oxaprozin
Flurbiprofen	Piroxicam
Indomethacin	Sulindac
Ketoprofen	Tolmetin
Ketorolac	

Interaction Summary

Concomitant use of gossypol with nonsteroidal antiinflammatory drugs (NSAIDs) such as ibuprofen may result in troublesome gastrointestinal distress and possible tissue damage.

Discussion

Tissue congestion, mucosal sloughing, necrosis of the mucosa, and hemorrhage of the intestinal wall have been associated with gossypol use.[1] Symptoms of nausea and appetite loss have led to the development of an enteric-coated preparation.[2] Considerably more study is needed in humans, but it is reasonable to as-

Rating Scale:
(1) Significant interaction
(2) Possibly significant interaction
(3) Interaction of relatively little significance
(4) Reported interaction that does not, in fact, exist or is insignificant

sume that concomitant use with NSAIDs might increase the risk of gastrointestinal side effects.

Management Suggestions

It is common for herbs and drugs to cause gastrointestinal side effects, however, the propensity of gossypol and NSAIDs to do so appears to exceed others. It would therefore be wise to avoid concomitant use.

NUTRIENTS—BILE ACID SEQUESTRANTS

RELATED DRUGS

Cholestyramine   Colestipol

POTENTIALLY IMPLICATED NUTRIENTS

Calcium   Iron
Folate   Vitamin A

Interaction Summary

Bile acid sequestrants have been reported to impair the absorption of numerous nutrients, including folate; vitamins A, B_{12}, E, and K; iron; and calcium.[1,2] However, the effect may not be clinically significant, and only folate supplementation may be needed for patients on long-term therapy with bile acid sequestrants.

Discussion

Cholestyramine was given over a period of 1 to 2.5 years to 18 children with familial hypercholesterolemia.[2] Prolonged treatment resulted in folate deficiency as demonstrated by decreased serum folate and a lowering of red blood cell folate. Dietary

---

Rating Scale:

(1) Significant interaction
(2) Possibly significant interaction

(3) Interaction of relatively little significance
(4) Reported interaction that does not, in fact, exist or is insignificant

folate (occurring primarily as anionic polyglutamates) tends to bind to cholestyramine resin, thus reducing folate absorption. Oral folic acid, 5 mg, overcame this depletion. Although cholestyramine interfered with the absorption of other nutrients, their levels remained in the normal range.

A study in rats administered cholestyramine also found decreased folate bioavailability.[1]

Management Suggestions

A folic acid supplement of 5 mg daily appears to be adequate to prevent folate depletion in patients taking bile acid sequestrants. The routine supplementation of fat-soluble vitamins appears unnecessary, though it may be advisable to monitor prothrombin time (a reflection of vitamin K status) and serum levels of vitamins A and E. On general principles, however, a comprehensive multivitamin-mineral supplement might be good insurance.

OMEPRAZOLE—
ST. JOHN'S WORT

Rating 2

RELATED DRUGS

Lansoprazole

Interaction Summary

The hypericin component of St. John's wort has been identified as a causative agent in the development of photosensitivity. Combination with proton pump inhibitors may increase this effect.

Discussion

Hypericin is a major ingredient in St. John's wort, often used for standardization purposes. It is also a known phototoxic agent.[1,2] One proposed mechanism for hypericin phototoxicity involves generation of free protons. Proton pump inhibitors may potentiate hypericin's phototoxic effects by decreasing intracellular pH.[3]

Management Suggestions

Although no case reports presently exist regarding the interaction of proton pump inhibitors with St. John's wort, clinicians should advise patients to avoid prolonged sun exposure when taking both.

Rating Scale:

(1) Significant interaction
(2) Possibly significant interaction

(3) Interaction of relatively little significance
(4) Reported interaction that does not, in fact, exist or is insignificant

ORAL CONTRACEPTIVES—
ANDROSTENEDIONE

Rating 3

RELATED DRUGS

Estradiol	Estropipate
Estrogen	Ethinyl estradiol

Interaction Summary

Androstenedione might increase estrogen-related side effects and risks in individuals taking estrogen.

Discussion

Androstenedione has become popular as a sports supplement, on the theory that it increases testosterone levels and improves athletic performance. However, there is no evidence that it is effective.[1] In addition, it appears more likely to elevate estrogen than testosterone levels.[2] This could increase estrogenic risks such as thromboembolism and breast and uterine cancer in individuals taking OCs or estrogen replacement therapy.

Management Suggestions

Women taking estrogen should avoid androstenedione.

Rating Scale:
(1) Significant interaction
(2) Possibly significant interaction
(3) Interaction of relatively little significance
(4) Reported interaction that does not, in fact, exist or is insignificant

ORAL CONTRACEPTIVES—
LICORICE

Rating 3

Interaction Summary

Licorice intake may exacerbate fluid retention experienced by some patients taking oral contraceptives. Patients may be at increased risk for elevated blood pressure as well.

Discussion

The active ingredient of licorice, glycyrrhizic acid, has been shown to inhibit 11-beta-hydroxysteroid dehydrogenase, an enzyme which metabolizes cortisol to cortisone.[1,2] In consequence, intrarenal levels of cortisol rise, causing inappropriate activation of mineralocorticoid receptors. The result is hypokalemia, edema, hypertension, decreased plasma renin, and decreased plasma aldosterone levels.[3]

Licorice (1.42, 2.84, 4.97, and 10.65 g/day) was administered for 4 weeks to four groups of 24 healthy subjects (12 males and 12 females) aged 22 to 39 years.[4] The plasma aldosterone concentration decreased from 35.8 ± 13.3 to 17.8 ± 8.3 pg/ml, $P = 0.04$ in the group receiving 10.65 g/day. Periorbital and ankle edema as well as weight gain was noted by the second week (63.4 $\pm$ 12.4 to 65.0 ± 12.5 kg body weight) for patients who were premenstrual or taking oral contraceptives.

Rating Scale:

(1) Significant interaction

(2) Possibly significant interaction

(3) Interaction of relatively little significance

(4) Reported interaction that does not, in fact, exist or is insignificant

Furthermore, hypokalemia and hypertension may be exacerbated in patients using both agents concomitantly. This occurred in a 21-year-old and a 36-year-old woman.[5] The latter patient also experienced pitting edema and pretibial edema. Hence concomitant use may prove troublesome for some patients taking oral contraceptives.

Management Suggestions

Patients taking oral contraceptives who are experiencing a mild increase in blood pressure and edema should be advised that licorice could worsen these side effects.

ORAL CONTRACEPTIVES—SOY

Interaction Summary

Based on presently available data, it appears unlikely that soy will interact with estrogenic drugs.

Discussion

Soy contains numerous phytoestrogens, including the isoflavones genistein and daidzen. However, some evidence suggests that it does not interact to a significant extent with oral contraceptives.

A study of 36 premenopausal women, of whom 20 were taking oral contraceptives, compared 2 months of normal diet to 2 months of diet supplemented with 38 mg of isoflavones.[1] No differences were seen in serum estrone, estradiol, sex hormone–binding globulin, dehydroepiandrosterone, prolactin, progesterone, menstrual cycle length, or urinary estrogen metabolites.

Management Suggestions

It is unlikely that dosage adjustments will need to be made when these two entities are used together.

Rating Scale:
(1) Significant interaction
(2) Possibly significant interaction

(3) Interaction of relatively little significance
(4) Reported interaction that does not, in fact, exist or is insignificant

ORAL CONTRACEPTIVES—
ST. JOHN'S WORT

Rating 2

NOTE: See Table I in Guengerich, 1999, for the most comprehensive list of CYP3A4 and p-glycoprotein drug substrates.[1]

RELATED DRUGS

Cyclosporine
CYP3A4 and
P-glycoprotein
drug substrates

HIV protease inhibitors
(e.g., saquinavir
and indinavir)

Interaction Summary

Concomitant use of St. John's wort extract causes increased metabolism of ethinylestradiol, the estrogenic component of oral contraceptives.

Discussion

Reliable case reports indicate that St. John's wort interferes with the effectiveness of oral contraceptives and has led to unwanted pregnancies.[2,3] The proposed mechanism is increased CYP3A4-dependent metabolism of the estrogenic component of the hormone preparations.

Rating Scale:
(1) Significant interaction
(2) Possibly significant interaction

(3) Interaction of relatively little significance
(4) Reported interaction that does not, in fact, exist or is insignificant

Management Suggestions

Reports to date suggest that St. John's wort compromises the estrogenic component of oral contraceptives, raising the risk of treatment failure.

ORALLY ADMINISTERED DRUGS—PSYLLIUM

Rating 1

OTHER POTENTIALLY IMPLICATED HERBS

Flaxseed

Ispaghula husk

Marshmallow leaf and root

Mullein

Psyllium seed husk

Interaction Summary

Psyllium may diminish absorption of orally administered drugs because of its mucilage content used as a stool-bulking agent.

Discussion

A 47-year-old woman had been stabilized on lithium with a corresponding blood level of 0.53 mmol/L.[1] Ispaghula husk (a psyllium hydrophilic mucilloid), 1 teaspoon in water twice daily, was initiated. Her lithium dose was increased (reason unspecified) to lithium citrate 10 ml twice daily, but 5 days after this dosage increase her lithium concentration decreased to 0.40 mmol/L. Three days later ispaghula was discontinued. Four days subsequently, a blood lithium concentration of 0.76 mmol/L was obtained. The temporal relationship strongly suggests that lithium absorption was impaired when given with this psyllium-related product.

Rating Scale:

(1) Significant interaction

(2) Possibly significant interaction

(3) Interaction of relatively little significance

(4) Reported interaction that does not, in fact, exist or is insignificant

Management Suggestions

Patients using herbal products with mucilage content should be advised to separate herb ingestion from the administration of oral medication by at least 2 hours in order to avoid impairment of the absorption of the medication.

PAROXETINE—
ST. JOHN'S WORT

Rating 2

RELATED DRUGS

Citalopram	Sertraline
Fluoxetine	Sumatriptan
Fluvoxamine	Tramadol
Nefazodone	Trazodone

OTHER POTENTIALLY IMPLICATED HERBS

Ayahuasca

Interaction Summary

Concomitant use of St. John's wort and selective serotonin re-uptake inhibitors (SSRIs) such as paroxetine may result in serotonin syndrome. The herb ayahuasca, which possesses alkaloids with MAO inhibitor action, may present a similar risk.

Discussion

St. John's wort appears to act similarly to SSRIs. In one study, researchers observed that St. John's wort extract caused down-regulation of serotonin receptors in cultured rat neuroblastoma cells.[1] Subchronic treatment in rodents has shown up-regulation

Rating Scale:
(1) Significant interaction
(2) Possibly significant interaction

(3) Interaction of relatively little significance
(4) Reported interaction that does not, in fact, exist or is insignificant

of 5-HT2 receptors in the frontal cortex.[2] Another study noted a 50% inhibition of synaptosomal uptake of serotonin, dopamine, and norepinephrine in mouse brain preparations at realistic concentrations of standard St. John's wort extracts.[3] This effect was found to correlate closely with hyperforin concentration in the herbal preparation.[4]

Based on these findings, concerns have arisen regarding the possible development of serotonin syndrome if St. John's wort is combined with SSRIs or other pharmaceuticals that can increase serotonin levels.

Serotonism is characterized by myoclonus, sweating, agitation, headache, abdominal pain, increased blood pressure, and hyperpyrexia. Combined use of paroxetine, 50 mg/day, and St. John's wort, 600 mg/day, resulted in weakness, fatigue, grogginess, and incoherence possibly due to serotonin syndrome.[5] The patient was arousable but had difficulty in getting out of bed. Her symptoms resolved spontaneously over the ensuing 2 hours.

Other reports strongly suggest that combining St. John's wort with sertraline, nefazodone, or trazodone also creates risk of serotonism.[6,7]

Serotonin syndrome can progress to acute delirium and has proven fatal.[8] Hence this possible drug-herb interaction needs to be taken very seriously.

The herb ayahuasca, a psychoactive beverage from the Amazon, contains harmala alkaloids with MAO inhibitor properties. One case report suggests that the combination of fluoxetine and ayahuasca caused the development of serotonin syndrome.[9]

Management Suggestions

Limited data suggest that St. John's wort should not be combined with SSRIs. If combined, the patient should be closely monitored for central nervous system depression, headache, sweating, and/or agitation. Keep in mind the long half-life of some SSRIs, including fluoxetine. The half-life of hyperforin (the leading candidate for active ingredient in St. John's wort) is thought to be about 9 hours.[10]

PENICILLAMINE—IRON

Rating 1

OTHER POTENTIALLY IMPLICATED SUPPLEMENTS

Copper	Ferrous sulfate
Ferrous fumarate	Iron polysaccharide
Ferrous gluconate	Zinc

Interaction Summary

Iron and other minerals may reduce the absorption of penicillamine. Conversely, mineral absorption may also be reduced.

Discussion

In a randomized crossover study of six healthy men, a single oral dose of penicillamine, 500 mg, was given after a dose of ferrous sulfate, 300 mg, and after an overnight fast.[1] The iron preparation reduced plasma levels of penicillamine to 35% of that after the fasting dose.

As penicillamine is thought to complex with iron, this interaction would be expected to reduce iron absorption as well.

Management Suggestions

Administer penicillamine at least 2 hours apart from iron preparations.

Rating Scale:
(1) Significant interaction
(2) Possibly significant interaction
(3) Interaction of relatively little significance
(4) Reported interaction that does not, in fact, exist or is insignificant

PENICILLAMINE—MAGNESIUM

Rating 2

Interaction Summary

Magnesium may reduce the absorption of penicillamine; magnesium absorption may also be reduced.

Discussion

In a randomized crossover study of six healthy men, a single oral dose of penicillamine, 500 mg, was given after a 30-ml dose of magnesium-containing antacid and also after an overnight fast.[1] Coadministration of the antacid reduced the plasma penicillamine level to 66% of that observed with the fasting dose of penicillamine. Though it was postulated that penicillamine complexed with magnesium, the antacid contained a combination of magnesium hydroxide and aluminum hydroxide, and no attempt was made to distinguish effects between the two.

Management Suggestions

Administer penicillamine at least 2 hours apart from magnesium preparations.

Rating Scale:
(1) Significant interaction
(2) Possibly significant interaction
(3) Interaction of relatively little significance
(4) Reported interaction that does not, in fact, exist or is insignificant

PENTOBARBITAL—EUCALYPTOL

Rating 2

RELATED DRUGS

Amobarbital	Methohexital
Aprobarbital	Phenobarbital
Butabarbital	Secobarbital
Mephobarbital	Thiopental

Interaction Summary

Eucalyptol may increase the metabolism of pentobarbital and other barbiturates, hence decreasing their effectiveness.

Discussion

Eucalyptol administered either subcutaneously or by aerosol increased liver metabolism of aminopyrine, p-nitro-anisol, and aniline in vitro and pentobarbital metabolism in vivo in rats.[1] In pharmacodynamics, pentobarbital-induced (25 mg/kg i.p.) sleep time in rats was approximately 50% less in rats given eucalyptol (19.6 ± 1 minutes) than in the control group (36.8 ± 2 minutes).[1] Hence, eucalyptol has demonstrated an ability to induce the metabolism of pentobarbital. It is likely that other drugs metabolized by the same liver microsomal enzymes will be affected in similar fashion. More study is needed as the pharmacologic effects of a wide range of drugs may be diminished by eucalyptol.

Rating Scale:
(1) Significant interaction
(2) Possibly significant interaction
(3) Interaction of relatively little significance
(4) Reported interaction that does not, in fact, exist or is insignificant

Management Suggestions

Patients should be advised to discontinue eucalyptol use (e.g., as an antiseptic agent or as an expectorant) prior to surgery when a barbiturate may be used. Patients who are not responding adequately to barbiturate therapy despite prior stabilization (e.g., phenobarbital for epilepsy) should be asked about recent use of agents known to induce liver microsomal enzymes, such as eucalyptol.

PENTOBARBITAL—VALERIAN

RELATED DRUGS

Amobarbital
Aprobarbital
Butabarbital

CNS depressants
(e.g., alcohol,
phenobarbital,
secobarbital)

OTHER POTENTIALLY IMPLICATED HERBS

Ashwagandha
Calendula
Catnip
Hops
Kava
Lady's slipper

Lemon balm
Passionflower
Sassafras
Skullcap
Yerba mansa

Interaction Summary

Valerian may potentiate the sedative effects of barbiturates such as pentobarbital.

Discussion

In a study designed to determine the pharmacologic profile of *Valeriana adscendens* in mice, it was found that locomotor activity and motor coordination were reduced and pentobarbital-

Rating Scale:
(1) Significant interaction
(2) Possibly significant interaction

(3) Interaction of relatively little significance
(4) Reported interaction that does not, in fact, exist or is insignificant

induced sleep was prolonged.[1] These effects were significant within 10 to 20 minutes of administration and were present for the duration of the 2-hour recording period.

Human studies are needed. These preliminary data suggest, however, that additive effects with pentobarbital can be expected.

Management Suggestions

If valerian is taken with a barbiturate such as pentobarbital, prolonged sleep is likely. Prudence dictates taking one or the other but not both simultaneously.

PHENELZINE—EPHEDRA

RELATED DRUGS

Isocarboxazid   Tranylcypromine

OTHER POTENTIALLY IMPLICATED HERBS

Black tea (caffeine content)   Scotch broom (tyramine
Green tea   content)
Guarana   Yohimbine
Mate

Interaction Summary

If used together, hypertensive crises may result.

Discussion

Ephedra refers to a family of plants containing 30 different species native to Asia, Mediterranean countries, and the United States.[1] The main alkaloids of ephedra are ephedrine and pseudoephedrine, whose metabolism is mediated by monoamine oxidases.[2] Inhibition of these enzymes by monoamine oxidase inhibitors (MAOIs) such as phenelzine may result in excessive ephedra-mediated effects such as hypertensive crises. Although there have not been any case reports, this interaction appears very likely based on the known pharmacologic action of the

---

Rating Scale:

(1) Significant interaction
(2) Possibly significant
     interaction

(3) Interaction of relatively little
     significance
(4) Reported interaction that
     does not, in fact, exist or is
     insignificant

agents involved. The German Commission E monographs also recognize the grave nature of this potential drug-herb interaction and recommend avoidance of concomitant use.

The herb Scotch broom contains tyramine, and for this reason a similar potential for interaction with MAOIs exists.[2] Numerous herbs contain caffeine and these too are problematic.

Given the increased use of MAOIs for atypical depression, clinicians need to assume vigilance for this drug-herb interaction.

Management Suggestions

Avoid concomitant use as hypertensive crises may occur.

PHENELZINE—GINSENG

Rating 2

RELATED DRUGS

Isocarboxazid   Tranylcypromine

Interaction Summary

According to two case reports, the combination of ginseng and phenelzine may cause insomnia, headache, and tremulousness.

Discussion

A 64-year-old woman reported insomnia, tremulousness, and headache after ingesting a ginseng-containing tea in addition to phenelzine.[1] She had drunk the tea previously, when not taking phenelzine, without consequence. Upon rechallenge with ginseng tea, the symptoms reappeared. A subsequent report detailed a 42-year-old woman who was taking phenelzine, 45 mg/day, for refractory depression.[2] The patient concurrently took ginseng. She noted a marked improvement in her mood, and became extremely active and optimistic, which was contrary to her previously introverted disposition. She invited strangers to her house for dinner and her sleep decreased, although she denied feeling tired. This patient had not previously experienced manic-like symptoms. Because she also began to experience irritability and tension headaches, she discontinued phenelzine. With the return of depressive symptoms, she was

---

Rating Scale:

(1) Significant interaction

(2) Possibly significant
     interaction

(3) Interaction of relatively little
     significance

(4) Reported interaction that
     does not, in fact, exist or is
     insignificant

restarted on phenelzine without ginseng, but had no therapeutic gain.

It has been found that ginsenosides inhibit cyclic AMP phosphodiesterase and thus perhaps augment the effects of monoamine oxidase inhibitors.[2,3] However, another potential explanation for such an interaction may be that some ginseng products reportedly also contain caffeine, a fact that is not listed on the label.[4]

Management Suggestions

Patients should avoid concomitant use of ginseng and phenelzine or any other MAOIs. Inactivation of phenelzine is via acetylation, with clinical effects persisting for up to 2 weeks following discontinuation of therapy; hence concomitant use should be avoided during this time period as well. Because the half-life of ginseng's relevant components is unknown, a recommendation based on this parameter cannot be offered.

PHENPROCOUMON—
ST. JOHN'S WORT

Rating 2

RELATED DRUGS

Anisindione   Warfarin
Dicumarol

Interaction Summary

St. John's wort may reduce plasma levels of drugs in the warfarin family.

Discussion

A single-blind, placebo-controlled study of 10 individuals found that St. John's wort significantly decreased the AUC of free phenprocoumon by 17.5% when taken at standard doses for 11 days.[1] Phenprocoumon was given in a single dose of 12 mg on day 11, and plasma concentrations were measured at intervals for 72 hours.

This report is currently available only in abstract form. The authors commented that phenprocoumon clearance may have been enhanced by induction of cytochrome P450 enzymes. However, no other evidence was presented nor was any single isoform implicated.

Rating Scale:
(1) Significant interaction
(2) Possibly significant interaction
(3) Interaction of relatively little significance
(4) Reported interaction that does not, in fact, exist or is insignificant

There are also seven case reports of individuals combining warfarin with St. John's wort, resulting in reduced anticoagulation as measured by INR.[2]

The metabolism of the coumarin anticoagulants is complex, with CYP2C9 being most closely linked to the metabolism of warfarin and phenprocoumon.[3] No work to date has suggested that St. John's wort induces this CYP isoform.

However, the R-form of warfarin (which possesses one-fourth the anticoagulant activity of the more potent S-form) is metabolized by CYP1A2 and both forms can be metabolized by CYP3A4.[4] Both of these CYP isoforms have shown to be induced by St. John's wort (see the **Cyclosporine—St. John's Wort, Indinavir—St. John's Wort,** and **Theophylline—St. John's Wort** articles); however, their role in the phenprocoumon interaction remains to be elucidated.

Management Suggestions

Individuals taking warfarin anticoagulants should have coagulation parameters measured if St. John's wort is taken concurrently.

PHENYTOIN—GINKGO

NOTE: This article refers to contaminants in ginkgo, not to ginkgo itself.

RELATED DRUGS

Carbamazepine	Mephenytoin
Gabapentin	Phenobarbital

Interaction Summary

Contaminants found in ginkgo preparations might diminish the anticonvulsant activity of phenytoin and related compounds.

Discussion

The neurotoxic ginkgotoxin 4'-O-methylpyridoxine has been found in the seeds of *Ginkgo biloba*.[1] This ginkgotoxin, an antivitamin B_6, interferes with amino acid metabolism and has been associated with convulsions and death in laboratory guinea pigs and mice.[1-3]

Ostensibly this neurotoxin should not be present in ginkgo preparations available for human use, since they are prepared from the leaves. However, in a recent study, this toxin was detected in leaves as well as in standardized ginkgo extracts

---

Rating Scale:

(1) Significant interaction
(2) Possibly significant interaction

(3) Interaction of relatively little significance
(4) Reported interaction that does not, in fact, exist or is insignificant

and was even detectable in homeopathic preparations.[4] 4'-O-methylpyridoxine was present in Tebonin Forte, Rokan, Daveri Forte, and Gingium in amounts of 8.13, 9.77, 3.8, and 7.18 μg/ml, respectively.

The highest amounts of ginkgolides were observed in late summer and early autumn coinciding with the maximum amount of ginkgotoxin in the leaves and seeds.[4] Fortunately, these amounts are considered nontoxic. However, given the lack of satisfactory standardization of herbal medicinals in the United States, it is conceivable that without regulation controlling contaminants, patients may be at risk from a batch with a high content of 4'-O-methylpyridoxine, depending on the season of harvest.

Management Suggestions

Preliminary evidence suggests that patients with epilepsy may be at risk for neurotoxic consequences if a ginkgo preparation with significant quantities of 4'-O-methylpyridoxine is ingested. With the present relative lack of regulation of these products, 4'-O-methylpyridoxine content is not under surveillance. Hence, patients who are stabilized on their current anticonvulsants could conceivably experience diminished control. More data are needed before concomitant use should be discouraged, but patients should be advised of this potential drug-herb interaction.

PHENYTOIN—SHANKHAPUSHPI

Interaction Summary

Shankhapushpi, an Ayurvedic herbal preparation advocated for the treatment of epilepsy, may decrease the effectiveness and lower the blood levels of phenytoin.

Discussion

Shankhapushpi is an Ayurvedic preparation containing *Convolvulus pluricaulis* (leaves), *Centella asiatica* (whole plant), *Nardostachys jatamansi* (rhizome), *Nepeta hinostana* (whole plant), *Nepeta elliptica* (whole plant), and *Onosma bracteatum* (leaves and flower). Although this preparation is advocated for the treatment of epilepsy, two patients previously stabilized on phenytoin lost seizure control.[1] Shankhapushpi administered as 1 teaspoonful three times daily decreased phenytoin levels from 9.62 ± 2.93 μmol/L to 5.10 ± 0.67 μmol/L ($P < 0.01$).

Additional study demonstrated that Shankhapushpi diminished phenytoin's antiepileptic effectiveness, as measured using maximal electroshock seizure. It is unknown if other anticonvulsants are similarly affected.

Management Suggestions

Avoid concomitant use of Shankhapushpi and phenytoin.

Rating Scale:
(1) Significant interaction
(2) Possibly significant interaction
(3) Interaction of relatively little significance
(4) Reported interaction that does not, in fact, exist or is insignificant

PHOSPHORUS—
ALUMINUM HYDROXIDE

Rating 1

OTHER POTENTIALLY IMPLICATED SUPPLEMENTS
Calcium

Interaction Summary

Aluminum-containing antacids can cause phosphorus depletion, especially with long-term use, and this can lead to calcium
depletion.

Discussion

The aluminum in aluminum-containing antacids combines with
phosphorus, rendering it unabsorbable.[1] That is the basis for the
use of aluminum hydroxide as a phosphate binder to treat hyperphosphatemia in hemodialysis patients. This interaction
leads to a loss of both phosphorus and calcium from bones.

One study found that prolonged administration of a commonly
used antacid containing aluminum and magnesium can produce
a phosphorus-depletion syndrome in healthy individuals.[2] Subjects included three normal volunteers, two patients with hy-
poparathyroidism, and one patient with pseudohypoparathy-
roidism. The phosphorus-depletion syndrome was characterized

Rating Scale:
(1) Significant interaction
(2) Possibly significant
     interaction

(3) Interaction of relatively little
     significance
(4) Reported interaction that
     does not, in fact, exist or is
     insignificant

by hypophosphatemia, hypophosphaturia, increased gastrointestinal calcium absorption, hypercalciuria, increased resorption of skeletal calcium and phosphorus, as well as anorexia, weakness, malaise, and bone pain.

At least one case has been reported in which antacid-induced phosphorus depletion was mistakenly diagnosed as primary hyperparathyroidism.[3]

In addition, as phosphorus levels become low in the blood and extracellular fluid, the body borrows phosphorus from bones to restore these levels. This starts the process of bone resorption, depleting bones of both calcium and phosphorus (as calcium phosphate). Osteomalacia (adult rickets) has also been reported to occur in such circumstances.

In these circumstances, increasing calcium intake to about 800 mg/day appears to help reduce calcium loss from bones.[1]

Management Suggestions

Long-term use of aluminum hydroxide as an antacid should probably be avoided. If aluminum hydroxide must be used, supplementation with calcium and phosphorus is recommended (milk might be useful for this purpose). Additionally, it may be advisable to administer the antacid 2 to 3 hours apart from meals or mineral supplements.

PIROXICAM—ST. JOHN'S WORT

RELATED DRUGS

ACE inhibitors
Amiodarone
Carbamazepine
Fluoroquinolones
Isotretinoin
Loop diuretics
Methotrexate
Methyldopa
NSAIDs
Oral contraceptives

Phenobarbital
Phenothiazines
Risperidone
Sulfonamides
Sulfonylureas
Tetracycline
Thiazide diuretics
Tricyclic antidepressants
Valproic acid

OTHER POTENTIALLY IMPLICATED HERBS

Dong quai

Interaction Summary

The hypericin component of St. John's wort has been identified as a causative agent in the development of photosensitivity. Combination with drugs with a known propensity to induce photosensitivity, such as piroxicam, may predispose the patient to severe reactions. Because of its furanocoumarin content, dong quai might also cause photosensitivity.

Rating Scale:
(1) Significant interaction
(2) Possibly significant interaction

(3) Interaction of relatively little significance
(4) Reported interaction that does not, in fact, exist or is insignificant

Discussion

The German Commission E Monographs advise that individuals ingesting St. John's wort should avoid excessive sun exposure, because this herb may cause photosensitization.[1] This effect has been observed in patients described as light-sensitive who took St. John's wort at twice the normal dose of 600 mg three times daily for 15 days.[2] In a study of 50 volunteers ingesting 600 mg of hypericum extract three times daily (daily doses of 5.6 mg total hypericin), increased sensitivity to UV light was observed.[3]

Photosensitivity was also noted in patients enrolled in a phase-1 AIDS trial who were intravenously administered high doses of synthetic hypericin.[4]

Phototoxicity has previously been observed in animals with a significant level of toxicity noted by day 7 and magnified by day 14, during continuous high intake of the herb.[5] Photosensitivity in livestock feeding on St. John's wort is well known.[6]

Combination of St. John's wort with drugs known to cause photosensitivity is a concern. No case reports yet exist documenting this interaction, but given the underlying toxicity profiles of both, it is a distinct possibility. Of particular concern is combining St. John's wort with drugs that have a long half-life, such as piroxicam.[7,8] If this herb-drug interaction is encountered, based on pharmacokinetic parameters, it could exist for several weeks.

Management Suggestions

Although no case reports presently exist regarding the interaction of St. John's wort with photosensitizing drugs, a clinician should advise patients to avoid prolonged sun exposure when taking both, and refer to complete lists of drug and herb photosensitizers.[9-13] Patients with AIDS are at particular risk given the high doses of St. John's wort sometimes advocated for antiviral activity. (This potential usage has been discredited.) In addition, these patients may be taking other medications which are known photosensitizers (e.g., trimethoprim/sulfamethoxazole).

PREDNISOLONE—LICORICE

RELATED DRUGS

Betamethasone

Dexamethasone

Hydrocortisone

Methylprednisolone

Prednisone

Triamcinolone

OTHER POTENTIALLY IMPLICATED HERBS

Magnolia officinalis

Perillae frutescens

Saiboku-To

Scutellaria baiclensis

Zizyphus vulgaris

Interaction Summary

Licorice may augment the effects of corticosteroids, such as prednisolone, through its ability to inhibit enzymatic metabolism of these drugs.

Discussion

The liver has two delta^4-reductase systems: a soluble delta^4-5-beta reductase and a microsomal delta^4-5-alpha reductase.[1] In human beings, 5-beta reductase predominates and is physiologically significant in the regulation and metabolism of cortisol and aldosterone.[1] Suppression of 5-beta reductase can be presumed to delay corticosteroid clearance and prolong the biological half-

Rating Scale:

(1) Significant interaction

(2) Possibly significant interaction

(3) Interaction of relatively little significance

(4) Reported interaction that does not, in fact, exist or is insignificant

life of cortisol. This mechanism leads to synergy between glucocorticoids and the glycyrrhetinic acid (GA) and glycyrrhizin (GL) found in licorice.[1]

In rat liver studies, both GA (50 mg/100 g) and GL (50 mg/100 g) (expressed as a percentage of the control for testosterone) significantly ($P < 0.001$) reduced delta^4-5-beta reductase (2.8% ± 1.7% and 57.2% ± 2.9%, respectively), aldosterone (5.0% ± 1.3% and 60.0% ± 2.9%, respectively), and cortisol (7.4% ± 5.1% and 75.0% ± 4.4%, respectively).[1] Further study demonstrated a similar effect on rat kidney 5-beta reductase.[2]

Chen et al. have undertaken pharmacokinetic studies to ascertain if glycyrrhizin affects prednisolone kinetics in human beings. Six healthy men were administered intravenous 0.075 mg/kg prednisolone (PSL) with or without 200 mg of GL.[3] GL significantly ($P < 0.05$) increased the area under the curve (AUC) from 126 ± 10 µg × hr/L to 199 ± 24 µg × hr/L and decreased clearance from 0.55 ± 0.02 L × kg/hr to 0.38 ± 0.05 L × kg/hr).[3] This was also demonstrated following oral administration of GL, where oral administration of 50 mg GL four times daily significantly ($P < 0.05$) increased free PSL AUC from 117 ± 27 to 182 ± 50 µg × hr/L and decreased clearance from 0.64 ± 0.16 to 0.42 ± 0.10 L × kg/hr.[4] The volume of distribution remained unchanged regardless of the route of administration.

This has translated into a potentiation of glucocorticoid effects when the drug is combined with GL in patients with rheumatoid arthritis or polyarteritis nodosa.[5] Rabbit studies have also confirmed an enhancing effect of GL on the immunosuppressive action of cortisone, as measured by circulating antibody in normal rabbits 10 days after immunization.[6]

A traditional Chinese herb combination called *Saiboku-To* has also been found to affect corticosteroid action by inhibiting 11-beta-hydroxysteroid dehydrogenase. It consists of *Perillae frutescens, Zizyphus vulgaris, Magnolia officinalis,* and *Scutellaria baiclensis.*[7]

Management Suggestions

When these agents are used concomitantly, the clinician should be aware that the effects of the corticosteroids may be enhanced and prolonged.

PRIMIDONE—NICOTINAMIDE

Rating 3

OTHER POTENTIALLY IMPLICATED SUPPLEMENTS
Niacin

Interaction Summary

Nicotinamide (niacinamide) may increase serum primidone levels.

Discussion

Nicotinamide is a supplemental form of niacin that does not possess the flushing side effect or lipid-lowering benefit of niacin. The addition of nicotinamide to primidone therapy in three children with seizure disorders decreased the conversion of primidone (PRM) to phenobarbital (PB), leading to decreased clearance and increased serum concentrations of primidone.[1]

Nicotinamide may inhibit CYP450 enzymes that metabolize primidone, leading to higher drug levels. The authors propose that increasing the PRM/PB ratio in this way and maintaining it at or above 1 may be desirable, because studies in mice show primidone to be significantly less neurotoxic than phenobarbital and yet similar in effect against electroshock seizures. For this reason, nicotinamide may be useful in poorly controlled or toxic patients with a low PRM/PB ratio.

Rating Scale:
(1) Significant interaction
(2) Possibly significant interaction

(3) Interaction of relatively little significance
(4) Reported interaction that does not, in fact, exist or is insignificant

Management Suggestions

Monitor serum primidone concentrations and adjust the primidone dose as needed or stop the nicotinamide. This interaction might be used beneficially in some cases.

PROCYCLIDINE—BETEL NUT

RELATED DRUGS

Benztropine	Donepezil
Bethanechol	Ethopropazine
Biperiden	Ipratropium
Dicyclomine	Tacrine
Diphenhydramine	Trihexyphenidyl

OTHER POTENTIALLY IMPLICATED HERBS

Jimson weed	Thorn apple
Mandrake	

Interaction Summary

The cholinergic activity of arecoline, an active alkaloid ingredient in betel nut, may offset the activity and decrease the efficacy of anticholinergic drugs such as procyclidine. Also, a potentiation effect might occur with cholinergic medications.

Discussion

Betel nut chewing has been associated with bronchoconstriction in 6 of 7 asthmatic patients and 1 of 6 healthy subjects, with one asthmatic patient showing a 30% decrease in FEV_1 150 minutes after chewing.[1] The authors attributed this effect to arecoline, a

---

Rating Scale:

(1) Significant interaction

(2) Possibly significant interaction

(3) Interaction of relatively little significance

(4) Reported interaction that does not, in fact, exist or is insignificant

cholinergic alkaloid constituent of betel nut. That only one of the healthy subjects experienced bronchoconstriction following betel nut exposure indicates that most healthy patients will not be adversely affected. However, asthmatic patients may be at risk. This interaction may be especially problematic for individuals with chronic obstructive pulmonary disease (COPD) or asthma who rely on ipratropium to maintain airway patency. However, no data exist exploring concomitant use.

Betel nut ingestion has also resulted in antipsychotic-induced movement disorders in patients previously controlled with an anticholinergic drug. A 51-year-old Indian man had been stabilized on fluphenazine decanoate, 50 mg depot every 3 weeks for the previous 2 years, and procyclidine, 5 mg twice daily.[2] He experienced marked rigidity, bradykinesia, and jaw tremor after 3 weeks of chewing betel nut, which resolved within 1 week of discontinuation of the herb. Another Indian patient, a 45-year-old man, had been maintained on flupenthixol, 60 mg depot every 2 weeks for 1 year.[2] After betel nut ingestion he developed marked stiffness, tremor, and akathisia that was unresponsive to dosage escalations of procyclidine of up to 20 mg daily. The movement disorders resolved within 4 days of discontinuation of betel nut ingestion. In each of these cases it is hypothesized that the anticholinergic effects of procyclidine were countered by the arecoline content of the betel nut.

Other potentially implicated herbs include jimson weed, mandrake, and thorn apple.[3]

Management Suggestions

These limited data suggest that betel nut is capable of offsetting the anticholinergic effects of procyclidine and perhaps related drugs. Patients who are taking both should be closely monitored because the beneficial effects of the anticholinergic drug (e.g., management of parkinsonism) may be markedly diminished.

PROPRANOLOL—BLACK PEPPER

Rating 1

RELATED DRUGS

Phenobarbital

Phenytoin

Rifampicin

Theophylline

Interaction Summary

When taken in relatively high doses or in formulations that deliberately concentrate the alkaloid piperine, black pepper may inhibit the metabolism and perhaps increase the absorption of several drugs. Although this can be used to therapeutic advantage in augmenting the pharmacologic effects of these drugs, it can also predispose the patient to an increased risk of side effects.

Discussion

Piperine is the major alkaloid component of black pepper and long pepper, which is used extensively in Ayurvedic formulations.[1] In a crossover study, six subjects received a single oral dose of propranolol 50 mg alone, theophylline 150 mg alone, or either in combination with piperine 20 mg daily for 7 days.[1] C_{max} increased from 45.0 (propranolol alone) to 92.0 ng/ml (propranolol plus piperine) with a similar increase in bioavail-

---

Rating Scale:

(1) Significant interaction

(2) Possibly significant interaction

(3) Interaction of relatively little significance

(4) Reported interaction that does not, in fact, exist or is insignificant

ability with the area under the curve (AUC) increasing from 561 to 1140 ng/ml/hr.[1]

Piperine was also associated with an increase in theophylline levels. C_{max} increased from 4.55 (theophylline alone) to 7.36 µg/ml (theophylline plus piperine) with an increase in bioavailability as measured by the AUC, which showed an increase from 43.8 to 85.7 µg/ml/hr.[1]

Phenytoin is affected in a similar fashion with an increase in C_{max} from 4.08 ± 0.21 (phenytoin alone) to 5.2 ± 0.4 µg/ml (phenytoin plus piperine).[2]

The bioavailability of rifampicin has also been enhanced with concomitant piperine administration.[3] The basis of this interaction is believed to result from piperine's ability to inhibit drug metabolism. Specifically, piperine has been found to inhibit arylhydrocarbon hydroxylation, ethylmorphine-N-demethylation, 7-ethoxycoumarin-O-deethylation, and 3-hydroxy-benzo(a) pyrene glucuronidation in rats.[4]

Piperine at 50 mg/kg and 80 mg/kg inhibited drug metabolizing enzymes in rats.[5] In particular, N,N^4-dimethyl amino benzaldehyde demethylase was 3.87 ± 0.13 nmol product formed/min/ mg protein (piperine 40 mg/kg) ($P < 0.05$) and 3.53 ± 0.25 (piperine 80 mg/kg) ($P < 0.02$) as compared to 4.37 ± 0.6 in controls (oil).[5] Maximal inhibition was noted at 1 hour and restored to normal within 6 hours.[4] Hence, it is conceivable that other drugs metabolized by the liver (which constitutes the majority of drugs) could be similarly affected.

It has also been proposed that piperine mediates changes in the biochemical milieu of the epithelial cells, resulting in stimulated absorptive ability of the intestine, and therefore in increased drug absorption.[3] This underlying mechanism could affect an even larger cadre of drugs.

Management Suggestions

Increased pharmacologic and adverse effects may be noted when propranolol is coadministered with piperine. Furthermore, drugs with a narrow therapeutic window that are liver metabolized (e.g., theophylline) should be monitored very closely if given concomitantly with piperine.

PROTEASE INHIBITORS
—GARLIC

Interaction Summary

Garlic supplements might interact unfavorably with protease inhibitors, reducing plasma levels as well as increasing risk of adverse effects.

Discussion

Two individuals with HIV experienced symptoms of gastrointestinal toxicity after combining ritonavir with garlic supplements.[1] Another study found evidence that garlic reduces plasma concentrations of saquinavir.[2]

Management Suggestions

Individuals taking protease inhibitors should avoid use of garlic supplements.

Rating Scale:
(1) Significant interaction
(2) Possibly significant interaction
(3) Interaction of relatively little significance
(4) Reported interaction that does not, in fact, exist or is insignificant

SAMe—LEVODOPA/CARBIDOPA

Rating 3

Interaction Summary

The drug levodopa may deplete endogenous SAMe. This may be responsible for some of the side effects of levodopa therapy, such as depression. However, exogenous SAMe might lead to loss of efficacy of levodopa therapy in Parkinson's disease.

Discussion

SAMe (*S*-adenosylmethionine) is a naturally occurring compound, derived from the amino acid methionine and the energy molecule adenosine triphosphate (ATP), that is used as a methyl donor in numerous biologic reactions. Conversion of dopa to dopamine in the brain is the basis for using levodopa (L-dopa) in Parkinson's disease (PD). As levodopa and its product dopamine are both avid methyl acceptors, it is thought that they may deplete brain levels of SAMe.[1,2]

One-half hour after injecting mice with levodopa, 100 mg/kg, brain levels of SAMe decreased by 64% and levels of the demethylated SAMe analog *S*-adenosylhomocysteine (SAH) increased by 89%, compared to saline control.[2] Subsequently, SAMe and SAH values returned to normal within 4 hours. A second experiment produced similar findings. Although dopamine levels increased as expected after levodopa administration, the data indicate that the increased methylation rate is

---

Rating Scale:

(1) Significant interaction

(2) Possibly significant interaction

(3) Interaction of relatively little significance

(4) Reported interaction that does not, in fact, exist or is insignificant

greater than the rate of dopamine accumulation, which could lead to a net decrease in dopamine.

In another animal study, injection of SAMe into the lateral ventricle caused tremors, rigidity, and hypokinesia as well as depletion of dopamine by as much as 50%.[3]

These are only short-term findings, but they suggest a possible hypothesis for the observed loss of efficacy of levodopa therapy over time: high levels of levodopa create greater demands for the methyl group, which depletes SAMe and stimulates the body to increase its production of SAMe.[2] This in turn accelerates the methylation and inactivation of levodopa and dopamine. In effect, levodopa brings about the destruction of both itself and dopamine.

The importance of these findings in humans is uncertain, but we do know that tolcapone, a COMT inhibitor used for Parkinson's disease, increases dopamine levels by preventing the methylation and inactivation of levodopa and dopamine.

These findings suggest that supplemental SAMe could increase the methylation/inactivation of L-dopa and dopamine, thus decreasing their therapeutic effect.

However, there is another perspective to consider. SAMe depletion by L-dopa could contribute to some of the side effects seen with L-dopa therapy, most notably depression. Depression is the most common mental disturbance in patients with Parkinson's disease, with a reported incidence as high as 46%, and L-dopa therapy is believed to contribute to it.[1] Because SAMe appears to have antidepressant activity, it is logical to wonder whether levodopa-induced reduction in SAMe levels contributes to the problem.

In a double-blind, placebo-controlled crossover study, SAMe, 400 mg, was given orally twice daily along with SAMe, 200 mg IM daily for 30 days, leading to significant improvement in depressive symptoms using the Hamilton Rating Scale for

Depression.[4] In this short-term study, SAMe did not appear to worsen symptoms of Parkinson's disease and did not require changes in levodopa therapy.

Management Suggestions

Until the possible long-term nature of this interaction is understood, it may be generally advisable to avoid combining SAMe supplements with levodopa. If SAMe is used to treat PD-associated depression in patients taking levodopa, monitor for worsening of PD symptoms.

SIMVASTATIN/NIACIN THERAPY—ANTIOXIDANTS

Rating 2

RELATED DRUGS

Atorvastatin	Lovastatin
Cerivastatin	Pravastatin
Fluvastatin	Simvastatin

Interaction Summary

Antioxidant therapy may impair the positive effects on HDL attributable to combined statin/niacin therapy.

Discussion

A 12-month study followed 153 subjects with coronary artery disease and low HDL levels.[1] Participants were randomized into four groups: simvastatin (10 to 20 mg) plus niacin (1 g bid); beta-carotene (12.5 mg bid), vitamin C (500 mg bid), vitamin E (400 IU bid), and selenium (50 μg bid); a combination of simvastatin-niacin and the antioxidants; or a placebo for all drugs. The results unexpectedly showed that while the simvastatin-niacin combination alone significantly elevated HDL levels, combined use of antioxidants with simvastatin-niacin markedly reduced this benefit. The cause of this interaction is not known.

Rating Scale:
(1) Significant interaction
(2) Possibly significant interaction
(3) Interaction of relatively little significance
(4) Reported interaction that does not, in fact, exist or is insignificant

Management Suggestions

Individuals taking niacin plus a statin drug with the goal of raising HDL levels should be advised to avoid high doses of antioxidants.

SPIRONOLACTONE—LICORICE

RELATED DRUGS

Amiloride   Triamterene

Interaction Summary

The effects of spironolactone may be diminished by coadministration of licorice. Conversely, spironolactone may offset the deleterious effects of excessive licorice intake.

Discussion

A 57-year-old woman who ingested 2 ounces of licorice daily for 2 years presented with hypertension, hypokalemic alkalosis, and electrocardiographic evidence of hypokalemia (potassium 2.7 mEq/L; normal: 3.5 to 5.0 mEq/L).[1] Institution of 1 g daily of oral spironolactone resulted in a fourfold increase in the sodium-potassium ratio in the urine, strongly negative sodium and strongly positive potassium balance, and correction of the hypokalemic alkalosis (pH = 7.40 during the fourth day of spironolactone administration; potassium: 4.4 mEq/L during the fifth day of spironolactone administration).[1] Licorice intake was maintained at 55 g/day during this observation.

Rating Scale:
(1) Significant interaction
(2) Possibly significant
     interaction

(3) Interaction of relatively little
     significance
(4) Reported interaction that
     does not, in fact, exist or is
     insignificant

The active ingredient of licorice, glycyrrhizic acid, has been shown to inhibit 11-beta-hydroxysteroid dehydrogenase, an enzyme which metabolizes cortisol to cortisone.[2,3] In consequence, intrarenal levels of cortisol rise, causing inappropriate activation of mineralocorticoid receptors. The result is hypokalemia, edema, hypertension, decreased plasma renin, and decreased plasma aldosterone levels.[4]

Licorice taken at 1.42, 2.84, 4.97, and 10.65 g/day was administered for 4 weeks to four groups of 24 healthy subjects (12 males and 12 females) aged 22 to 39 years.[5] The plasma aldosterone concentration decreased from 35.8 ± 13.3 to 17.8 ± 8.3 pg/ml ($P = 0.04$) in the group receiving 10.65 g/day.

Based on this physiological effect, it is reasonable to assume that long-term use of high doses of licorice could counteract the effects of spironolactone.

Management Suggestions

Licorice added to established therapy with spironolactone may result in a diminished response to spironolactone. The two agents should not be used together unless spironolactone is administered to treat licorice toxicity.

STATIN DRUGS—NIACIN

Rating 2

RELATED DRUGS

Atorvastatin	Lovastatin
Cerivastatin	Pravastatin
Fluvastatin	Simvastatin

Interaction Summary

The addition of niacin to statin therapy improves HDL levels. Concerns about increased risk of myopathy and rhabdomyolysis have been reduced by the results of recent studies.

Discussion

Lovastatin therapy is associated with a relatively small risk of myopathy. At one time, myopathy was reported to occur in up to 5% of patients taking lovastatin and high-dose niacin together. Since then, however, controlled trials using statin drugs with niacin have reported few or no cases of myopathy, so the actual incidence of myopathy with this combination is probably lower than previously thought.[1,3] The risk may be primarily confined to individuals with impaired kidney function.[1] A recent study confirms the safety as well as benefits of a once-daily niacin-lovastatin formulation.[2] This ongoing, 1-year, multicenter, open-label study used an initial dose of 500 mg niacin/10 mg lovastatin, which has been increased to 1000/20, 1500/30, and

---

Rating Scale:

(1) Significant interaction

(2) Possibly significant interaction

(3) Interaction of relatively little significance

(4) Reported interaction that does not, in fact, exist or is insignificant

2000/40 at monthly intervals, if tolerated. No cases of myopathy have been observed thus far. The incidence of elevated liver enzymes greater than three times the upper limit has been less than 1%.

One study found that even a low dose of niacin (100 mg) added to statin therapy raises HDL levels.[4]

Management Suggestions

If symptoms of myopathy, such as unusual muscle pain or weakness, occur in a patient taking niacin and a statin drug, measure plasma CK (creatine kinase) levels to confirm the diagnosis. Discontinuation of drug therapy should resolve the problem.

TAMOXIFEN—TANGERETIN

Interaction Summary

Tangeretin, a citrus flavonoid present in tangerines, may interfere with the effectiveness of tamoxifen.

Discussion

In vitro, tangeretin shows effects similar to tamoxifen in suppressing human mammary cancer cells, and a combination of the two shows additive benefits.[1]

Surprisingly, however, the opposite effect was found when researchers tried to confirm the promising in vitro findings with an in vivo study in mice that were deliberately injected with human mammary cancer cells.[2] Eighty female nude mice were inoculated subcutaneously with human MCF-7/6 mammary adenocarcinoma cells. Groups of 20 mice were treated orally by adding the following substances to their drinking water: tamoxifen (30 µmol), tangeretin (100 µmol), tamoxifen plus tangeretin (30 µmol plus 100 µmol), or solvent. The tamoxifen treatment resulted in a statistically significant inhibition of tumor growth compared to solvent treatment (two-sided $P = 0.001$). Tangeretin treatment failed to inhibit tumor growth, while the tamoxifen plus tangeretin combination completely neutralized tamoxifen's inhibitory effect. Median survival time of mice treated with tamoxifen plus tangeretin was reduced compared to that of

---

Rating Scale:

(1) Significant interaction

(2) Possibly significant interaction

(3) Interaction of relatively little significance

(4) Reported interaction that does not, in fact, exist or is insignificant

mice treated with tamoxifen alone (14 versus 56 weeks; two-sided $P = 0.002$). Tangeretin (1 μmol or higher) inhibited the cytolytic effect of murine natural killer cells on MCF-7/6 cells in vitro, and this may explain why tamoxifen's benefit was abolished in the presence of tangeretin.

Management Suggestions

Whether tangeretin might exert similar effects on tamoxifen in humans is not known; however, based on these preliminary findings, it would seem advisable to counsel against excessive intake of tangeretin during tamoxifen therapy.

TETRACYCLINES—IRON

RELATED DRUGS

Demeclocycline

Doxycycline

Methacycline

Minocycline

Oxytetracycline

Tetracycline

OTHER POTENTIALLY IMPLICATED SUPPLEMENTS

Calcium

Magnesium

Zinc

Interaction Summary

Numerous metallic mineral salts bind with tetracycline antibiotics and interfere with their absorption, potentially resulting in diminished antibiotic efficacy. Mineral absorption is likewise reduced. Minerals known to interact with tetracyclines include calcium, magnesium, iron, and zinc. Other minerals may also interact.

Discussion

Tetracyclines form insoluble chelates with polyvalent metal cations including iron, calcium, magnesium, and zinc.[1] The result is reduced absorption of both the antibiotic and mineral.

Rating Scale:

(1) Significant interaction

(2) Possibly significant interaction

(3) Interaction of relatively little significance

(4) Reported interaction that does not, in fact, exist or is insignificant

In one study, ferrous sulfate (40 mg elemental iron) reduced serum levels of tetracycline and oxytetracycline significantly more than methacycline and doxycycline, compared to control (without iron).[1]

The severity of an interaction depends on the particular tetracycline derivative and formulation of the cation, the doses, dosing schedules, and pharmaceutical factors. For instance, ferrous sulfate capsules may reduce tetracycline absorption more than tablets, while enteric-coated iron preparations reduce absorption less than regular tablets. The interference also appears to be less with sustained-release iron formulations. Both ferrous and ferric iron bind with tetracycline, with the ferric form binding stronger.[2] In one study, coadministration of 200 mg of ferrous sulfate caused plasma levels of tetracycline to drop by approximately 50% and levels of some tetracycline derivatives to decrease by as much as 80% to 90%. Taking iron 3 hours before or 2 hours after the antibiotic prevented the problem.

Conversely, tetracycline interferes with iron absorption. One study found substantial decreases in iron absorption (30% to 40%) in individuals with either normal or depleted iron stores when tetracycline, 500 mg, was given simultaneously with 50 mg of ferrous iron.[3]

Milk (being calcium-rich) inhibits the absorption of tetracycline, doxycycline, and oxytetracycline, but serum concentrations of these antibiotics appear to remain in the therapeutic range.[1] Milk's effects on methacycline and demeclocycline appear to be more substantial.

Similar interactions have been reported with zinc.[4,5] Antacids containing aluminum, magnesium, or calcium have been found to substantially decrease the absorption of all tetracyclines.[1]

Management Suggestions

Administer tetracyclines 3 to 4 hours apart from milk and dairy products containing calcium and from supplements containing metallic cations.

THEOPHYLLINE—IPRIFLAVONE

Rating 1

RELATED DRUGS

Aminophylline	Phenytoin
Dyphylline	Tolbutamide
Oxtriphylline	Warfarin

Interaction Summary

Through CYP interactions, ipriflavone might increase serum levels of theophylline and other drugs metabolized by CYP1A2 or CYP2C9, thereby causing a risk of toxicity.

Discussion

Ipriflavone, a synthetic isoflavone that inhibits bone resorption, is used to treat osteoporosis. Evidence suggests that ipriflavone may inhibit certain CYP liver enzymes, and this may lead to increased serum levels of some drugs.

In an in vitro study, the researchers measured inhibition of theophylline biodegradation in human liver microsomes by different concentrations of ipriflavone or its metabolites MI, 7-hydroxy-isoflavone, and MV, 7-(1-carboxy-ethoxy)-isoflavone.[1] The results suggest that enzymatic degradation of theophylline is inhibited by ipriflavone and its metabolites MI and MV. A comprehensive in vitro study was then performed to analyze

---

Rating Scale:

(1) Significant interaction

(2) Possibly significant interaction

(3) Interaction of relatively little significance

(4) Reported interaction that does not, in fact, exist or is insignificant

the effect of ipriflavone on the cytochrome P450 family of enzymes.[2] Seven isoforms of the P450 enzyme were evaluated for inhibition by ipriflavone and its metabolites MI and MV. The most abundant metabolite, MV, did not inhibit any of the P450 isozymes. Ipriflavone and its metabolite MI inhibited the isozyme CYP1A2. Besides theophylline, this could affect the metabolism of caffeine, theobromine, and other polycyclic aromatic compounds.

Reduced theophylline clearance and increased serum levels were found in a patient with chronic obstructive pulmonary disease who was taking a combination of theophylline and ipriflavone.[3] After ipriflavone withdrawal, serum theophylline concentrations decreased to levels similar to those found before ipriflavone administration. Although there was no clinical evidence of theophylline toxicity in this case, this finding is of concern, since ipriflavone might be used by asthmatic patients receiving long-term steroid therapy in hopes of preventing or treating iatrogenic osteoporosis.

Inhibition of the CYP2C9 isozyme was also observed in the in vitro study just described. This could lead to interactions with such drugs as tolbutamide, phenytoin, and warfarin, among others. These interactions are difficult to predict based on in vitro studies because steady state drug concentrations and the amount of active drug at the enzyme site in vivo may be less than in vitro.[2] However, they raise concerns similar to those regarding theophylline: both warfarin and phenytoin contribute to osteoporosis. The use of ipriflavone to prevent or treat iatrogenic osteoporosis could result in higher serum levels of these drugs, with potentially serious consequences.

Management Suggestions

Individuals taking any potentially affected drugs should be advised to use ipriflavone only under close physician supervision.

THEOPHYLLINE—
ST. JOHN'S WORT

Rating 2

RELATED DRUGS

Clomipramine   Imipramine
Clozapine   Olanzapine

Interaction Summary

St. John's wort may stimulate the metabolism of theophylline, resulting in greater dosage requirements for theophylline. However, abrupt discontinuation of St. John's wort by a patient stabilized on theophylline may lead to toxic, supratherapeutic theophylline levels. Similar interactions may occur with clomipramine, clozapine, imipramine, and olanzapine.

Discussion

In a single case report, a 42-year-old woman is described who required relatively high doses of theophylline (Theo-Dur, 800 mg twice daily) to maintain a theophylline blood level of 9.2 μg/ml.[1] She had been stabilized on theophylline, 300 mg twice daily, for several months, taken concomitantly with other medications including albuterol, amitriptyline, furosemide, ibuprofen, inhaled triamcinolone acetonide, morphine, potassium, prednisone, valproic acid, zafirlukast, and zolpidem. The only new addition to her medication regimen had been the initiation

Rating Scale:

(1) Significant interaction
(2) Possibly significant
    interaction

(3) Interaction of relatively little
    significance
(4) Reported interaction that
    does not, in fact, exist or is
    insignificant

of St. John's wort, 300 mg/day (standardized to 0.3% hypericin), initiated 2 months before this evaluation.

On her own volition, the patient discontinued St. John's wort after noting the temporal relationship between its introduction into her regimen and the subsequent problems with her theophylline levels. Her theophylline concentration 7 days after discontinuation of St. John's wort was 19.6 µg/ml. Her theophylline dosage was then adjusted downward.

The authors propose that induction of hepatic enzymes occurred, specifically induction of cytochrome P450 CYP1A2 mediated by a transcriptional enhancer sequence known as xenobiotic response element (XRE). Nebel et al. have begun to investigate the mechanistic basis for this potential metabolic interaction between the components of St. John's wort and theophylline. Preliminary results indicated 1.8-fold induction of XRE at 12.5 µM hypericin to 5.20-fold induction at 125 µM hypericin as compared to untreated controls.[1]

While CYP1A2 is not one of the more quantitatively important cytochrome P450s, it does metabolize other important drugs whose clearance may be theoretically increased as well. These drugs include clomipramine and imipramine, two older tricyclic antidepressants, and clozapine and olanzapine, two newer antipsychotic drugs.

Management Suggestions

Given the narrow therapeutic window of theophylline, concomitant use of St. John's wort should be avoided until this drug-herb interaction has been better characterized. Hopefully, with the diminishing use of theophylline and the tricyclic antidepressants (clomipramine and imipramine), this interaction will only rarely be encountered.

More important is the potential for increased clearance of the newer antipsychotic drugs, clozapine and olanzapine, in schizophrenic patients. The addition of St. John's wort to regimens of patients on either drug might cause breakthrough psychotic episodes as a result of increased drug clearance. Conversely, patients who are stabilized on either of these drugs *while already using* St. John's wort should not injudiciously stop taking the herb without the advice of their physician[2] (the discontinuation of the CYP-inducer can potentially cause clozapine or olanzapine drug concentrations to rise to toxic levels). This is particularly serious in the case of clozapine, which can predispose patients to seizures and agranulocytosis.

THYROID HORMONE—CALCIUM

Rating 1

RELATED DRUGS

Dextrothyroxine   Liotrix
Levothyroxine   Thyroglobulin
Liothyronine

Interaction Summary

Evidence suggests that calcium carbonate may interfere with the absorption of levothyroxine, possibly posing a risk of hypothyroidism.

Discussion

A 49-year-old woman taking levothyroxine, 150 μg/day, reported headache, dizziness, mood changes, depression, and lethargy.[1] Hypothyroidism was suspected and confirmed by an initial TSH of 21.85 IU/ml (normal: 0.35 to 5.5 IU/ml) and elevated TSH on repeated measurement. She admitted to concurrent ingestion of the thyroid medication with a commonly used calcium carbonate product (3 tablets daily) for osteoporosis prevention. The patient was instructed to separate administration times of supplement and drug and follow-up revealed a TSH of 3.31 IU/ml. Other case reports describe this same possible interaction,[1,2] with the proposed mechanism being de-

---

Rating Scale:

(1) Significant interaction

(2) Possibly significant interaction

(3) Interaction of relatively little significance

(4) Reported interaction that does not, in fact, exist or is insignificant

creased absorption of levothyroxine resulting from chelation by calcium carbonate.

A prospective cohort study has validated these case reports.[3] Twenty individuals with hypothyroidism on long-term, stable-dose levothyroxine were included in the study. Participants were given calcium carbonate supplying 1200 mg/day of elemental calcium for 3 months, and then followed for 2 months after discontinuing calcium carbonate. The results showed a significant reduction in mean free T(4) and total T(4) levels during the calcium period, which increased after calcium was discontinued. The values reported in the study were as follows: mean free T(4) levels were 17 pmol/L (1.3 ng/dl) at baseline, 15 pmol/L (1.2 ng/dl) during calcium treatment, and 18 pmol/L (1.4 ng/dl) after calcium discontinuation (overall $P < 0.001$); mean total T(4) levels were 118 nmol/L (9.2 μg/dl) at baseline, 111 nmol/l (8.6 μg/dl) during calcium treatment, and 120 nmol/L (9.3 μg/dl) after calcium discontinuation (overall $P = 0.03$). Mean thyrotropin levels rose significantly, from 1.6 mIU/L at baseline to 2.7 mIU/L during calcium treatment, and fell to 1.4 mIU/L after calcium was discontinued.

Management Suggestions

Calcium supplements are commonly taken for prevention of osteoporosis; patients on thyroid medication should be instructed to take the drug and calcium supplements at different times of the day. Consider monitoring thyroid parameters to ensure euthyroid status.

THYROID HORMONE—
CARNITINE

Rating 3

RELATED DRUGS

Dextrothyroxine   Liotrix
Levothyroxine   Thyroglobulin
Liothyronine

Interaction Summary

Evidence suggests that supplemental carnitine partially blocks
the action of thyroid hormone.

Discussion

In vitro studies suggest that carnitine is a peripheral antagonist
of TH action, acting at or before the nuclear envelope.[1]

A 6-month, double-blind trial evaluated the effects of L-carnitine
in 50 women with benign nodular goiter who were taking exogenous T_4 to suppress TSH.[2] Participants received either
placebo or carnitine at a dose of 2 or 4 g daily. The results showed
significantly greater reductions on a 5-point scale designed to
quantify subjective and objective symptoms of hyperthyroidism
in both carnitine groups as compared to the placebo group. In
addition, biochemical markers indicated significantly less bone
demineralization in the carnitine group as compared to the

Rating Scale:
(1) Significant interaction
(2) Possibly significant
     interaction

(3) Interaction of relatively little
     significance
(4) Reported interaction that
     does not, in fact, exist or is
     insignificant

placebo group. The two doses of carnitine produced similar effects.

Management Suggestions

Carnitine supplements should be regarded with caution when used among individuals prescribed exogenous thyroid hormone.

THYROID HORMONE—IRON

RELATED DRUGS

Dextrothyroxine
Levothyroxine
Liothyronine

Liotrix
Thyroglobulin

RELATED SUPPLEMENTS

Ferrous fumarate
Ferrous gluconate

Ferrous sulfate
Iron polysaccharide

Interaction Summary

Iron salts may impair the effect of levothyroxine, probably by forming a complex with the thyroid hormone and decreasing its absorption.

Discussion

Iron is believed to form a complex with levothyroxine and reduce its absorption. A trial involving 14 patients with primary hypothyroidism found that ferrous sulfate impaired the effect of levothyroxine when the two were given concurrently.[1] Patients were given ferrous sulfate, 300 mg, and levothyroxine, 0.075 to 0.15 mg, together each morning 30 to 60 minutes before breakfast. At week 12, thyroid stimulating hormone (TSH) had in-

---

Rating Scale:

(1) Significant interaction
(2) Possibly significant interaction

(3) Interaction of relatively little significance
(4) Reported interaction that does not, in fact, exist or is insignificant

creased from 1.6 to 5.4 mU/L in 11 patients, compared to base-line. TSH concentrations in one patient increased from 2.6 to 40.8 mU/L. TSH serum concentrations were high enough to indicate hypothyroidism in two patients, and the clinical hypothyroidism score increased in nine patients.

Management Suggestions

Administer iron salts as far apart as possible from levothyroxine. Monitor thyroid function and adjust the dose of levothyroxine as needed.

THYROID HORMONE—SOY

Rating 2

RELATED DRUGS

Dextrothyroxine
Levothyroxine
Liothyronine

Liotrix
Thyroglobulin

Interaction Summary

Soy and soy-derived products may interfere with thyroid hormone absorption and thyroid function.

Discussion

Soy formula may interfere with the absorption of thyroid medication in infants.[1] Additionally, soy may directly interfere with thyroid function.[2,3] The result may be a need to increase the infant's dosage of thyroid medication. However, if infant soy formula is then discontinued, the thyroid dosage may need to be decreased.

Management Suggestions

Based on these findings, individuals with impaired thyroid function should use soy (e.g., soybeans, soy milk, tofu) with caution.

Rating Scale:
(1) Significant interaction
(2) Possibly significant interaction

(3) Interaction of relatively little significance
(4) Reported interaction that does not, in fact, exist or is insignificant

TRIMETHOPRIM-SULFAMETHOXAZOLE—PABA

Rating 2

RELATED DRUGS

Dapsone (DDS)   Sulfones
Sulfonamides

Interaction Summary

The antimicrobial effects of sulfonamides and sulfones may be impaired by supplementation with para-aminobenzoic acid (PABA).

Discussion

Microorganisms that must synthesize their own folic acid are susceptible to certain sulfones and sulfonamides, which appear to work by competitively displacing PABA from its binding site on an enzyme that catalyzes a key step in the biosynthesis of folic acid.[1] For this reason, PABA supplementation may reverse the antimicrobial action of these agents.

Investigations involving human volunteers subjected to mosquito-induced infections found that the antimalarial effects of the sulfone dapsone (DDS) were impaired by PABA supplementation.[2] Either dapsone alone or dapsone in combination

---

Rating Scale:
(1) Significant interaction
(2) Possibly significant
     interaction

(3) Interaction of relatively little
     significance
(4) Reported interaction that
     does not, in fact, exist or is
     insignificant

with PABA was given to 39 volunteers not previously exposed to malaria, and then the subjects were bitten by infected mosquitos. Infection was suppressed in 19 of 23 volunteers given dapsone, 25 mg and 50 mg daily, beginning before exposure to infected mosquitos and continuing 1 month after exposure. In contrast, all five volunteers given PABA, 4 g/day (1 g every 6 hours), and dapsone, 25 mg/day, beginning on the day before being bitten suffered acute attacks of malaria.

Management Suggestions

It may be advisable for patients taking sulfonamides or sulfones to avoid PABA supplements.

TRIMETHOPRIM-SULFAMETHOXAZOLE—POTASSIUM

Rating 3

Interaction Summary

Combining potassium with trimethoprim-sulfamethoxazole (TMP-SMZ) therapy may cause hyperkalemia.

Discussion

Hyperkalemia is known to occur with high-dose trimethoprim in patients with AIDS. A study of hospitalized patients treated for various infections found that standard-dose TMP-SMZ could also lead to hyperkalemia.[1] Of 80 patients treated with TMP-SMZ, 62.5% developed serum potassium concentrations greater than 5.0 mmol/L, and 21.2% developed severe hyperkalemia (serum potassium ≥ 5.5 mmol/L). The 25-patient control group in this study, treated with other antibiotics, showed a modest decrease in potassium concentrations.

Trimethoprim is structurally similar to the potassium-sparing diuretic amiloride, which inhibits distal tubule sodium reabsorption and potassium secretion, and this is thought to be the probable mechanism for the development of hyperkalemia.

Given this effect, individuals taking trimethoprim should avoid potassium supplements. Symptoms of hyperkalemia include

---

Rating Scale:
(1) Significant interaction
(2) Possibly significant interaction

(3) Interaction of relatively little significance
(4) Reported interaction that does not, in fact, exist or is insignificant

cardiac arrhythmias, muscle weakness, nausea, vomiting, irritability, and diarrhea.

Management Suggestions

Question patients to determine whether they might be ingesting a high-potassium diet or taking a potassium supplement, salt substitute containing potassium, or potassium-sparing diuretic. Monitor serum potassium concentrations and adjust potassium intake as needed.

VERAPAMIL—CALCIUM

RELATED DRUGS

Amlodipine   Felodipine
Bepridil   Isradipine
Diltiazem

OTHER POTENTIALLY IMPLICATED SUPPLEMENTS
Vitamin D

Interaction Summary

Calcium salts may antagonize some of the effects of calcium channel blockers. Most of the evidence relates to calcium infusion; however, oral calcium (especially when combined with vitamin D) might produce a similar effect.

Discussion

Calcium channel blockers inhibit the normal movement of extracellular calcium ions across the cell membrane and into myocardial cells and vascular and GI smooth muscle. This "calcium-blocking" effect decreases mechanical contraction of the heart and smooth muscle and results in improved blood flow and oxygen to the heart, dilation of peripheral arteries, and decreased total peripheral resistance, blood pressure, and afterload. Calcium infusion may antagonize some of these effects;

Rating Scale:
(1) Significant interaction
(2) Possibly significant interaction
(3) Interaction of relatively little significance
(4) Reported interaction that does not, in fact, exist or is insignificant

oral supplementation with calcium plus vitamin D might also produce some similar effects.

In dogs, calcium chloride given by infusion reversed some of verapamil's effects in a dose-related manner.[1] Average serum calcium levels of 6.5 mEq/L reversed verapamil-induced depressive effects on cardiac output and blood pressure, but did not affect verapamil's prolongation of AH intervals and slowing of the sinus rate. Increasing serum calcium to 8.2 mEq/L significantly shortened AH intervals but still had no effect on sinus rate or AV block.

Interestingly, a study of rabbit AV nodal preparations suggests that, in some cases, IV calcium–induced hypercalcemia may potentiate, rather than counteract, verapamil's depression of AV nodal conduction.[2]

Calcium infusion has been used clinically to counteract effects of verapamil, such as hypotension,[3,4] and as a treatment for verapamil overdose,[5,6] with mixed results.

A chart review of patients who had received IV verapamil for supraventricular tachydysrhythmias and pretreatment with low-dose calcium chloride (providing 27 mg or less of ionized calcium) found calcium was effective in counteracting verapamil-induced hypotension, particularly in patients who presented with low blood pressure.[7]

One study suggests that a single dose of calcium gluconate may not be effective in counteracting the blood pressure–lowering effect of verapamil.[8] In 20 hypertensive patients on long-term verapamil therapy, a single infusion of calcium gluconate (1375 mg) did not change average blood pressure or heart rate, though blood pressure did fall significantly in a few individual patients.

Vitamin D potentiates the effects of oral calcium by increasing its absorption and utilization. A patient whose atrial fibrillation had been successfully treated with verapamil began taking oral supplements of calcium and high-dose calciferol (a form of vitamin D) for osteoporosis.[9] A week later, atrial fibrillation reappeared and was reconverted to sinus rhythm by IV administration of verapamil and fluids.

Management Suggestions

Administration of IV calcium salts may be used therapeutically to reverse some of the cardiac depressant effects of verapamil and possibly other calcium channel blockers. Conversely, patients on calcium channel blockers who take calcium or vitamin D supplements should be closely monitored for reduced effectiveness of the treatment.

VITAMIN A—VALPROIC ACID

Rating 2

RELATED DRUGS

Barbiturates	Phenobarbital
Carbamazepine	Phenytoin
Divalproex sodium	Primidone
Ethosuximide	Valproate sodium

Interaction Summary

Valproic acid and other anticonvulsants increase the risk of birth defects, perhaps by altering endogenous retinoid metabolism. It is possible that coadministration with supplemental vitamin A could increase this risk.

Discussion

Anticonvulsants as a class have been associated with teratogenic effects when administered during pregnancy. The numerous proposed mechanisms include one involving the effects of these drugs on vitamin A (retinol) metabolism.

Vitamin A and its metabolites, especially all-*trans* retinoic acid, play a significant role in many embryonic development processes. Both excess and deficiency of vitamin A have been associated with teratogenic effects and alterations in related plasma retinoids might also be harmful.

Rating Scale:

(1) Significant interaction

(2) Possibly significant interaction

(3) Interaction of relatively little significance

(4) Reported interaction that does not, in fact, exist or is insignificant

One study involving 75 infants and children taking various anticonvulsant agents and 29 untreated controls found significant alterations in the levels of retinol and some isomers and oxidative metabolites of retinoic acid.[1] Valproic acid monotherapy, in particular, increased retinol levels in the young age group. Conversely, plasma levels of two oxidative metabolites of retinoic acid were strongly decreased in all patient groups treated with phenytoin, phenobarbital, carbamazepine, and ethosuximide, in combination with valproic acid, compared to controls.

These effects on endogenous retinoid metabolism may be related to the teratogenesis observed with anticonvulsant agents.

Whether combining vitamin A and anticonvulsants increases the risk of teratogenesis, however, remains unclear.

Management Suggestions

Although this risk is hypothetical, it might be advisable to avoid coadministration of anticonvulsants and vitamin A during early pregnancy.

VITAMIN B$_1$ (THIAMINE)— LOOP DIURETICS

Rating 2

RELATED DRUGS

Bumetanide   Furosemide

Ethacrynic acid   Torsemide

Interaction Summary

Loop diuretics as well as other factors may contribute to vitamin B$_1$ (thiamine) deficiency in patients with congestive heart failure (CHF).

Discussion

Thiamine deficiency has been reported to occur in 20% of CHF patients who were treated with loop diuretic therapy, presumably due to increased urinary loss of the vitamin.[1] This thiamine depletion may be a factor in impaired cardiac function in patients with CHF.

In one small study, patients with chronic CHF receiving furosemide, 80 to 240 mg, for 3 to 14 months were compared to age-matched patients without heart failure and not taking diuretics.[1] A thiamine deficiency was found in 21 of the 23 furosemide-treated patients compared to 2 of the 16 controls. This finding in the presence of high urinary thiamine excretion

---

Rating Scale:

(1) Significant interaction

(2) Possibly significant interaction

(3) Interaction of relatively little significance

(4) Reported interaction that does not, in fact, exist or is insignificant

appeared to exclude the possibility that decreased thiamine intake or absorption caused the deficiency. More likely, the cause was an excessive urinary loss of thiamine caused by furosemide in the presence of CHF, or the combined effects of furosemide and CHF on the kidneys. A 7-day course of IV thiamine, 100 mg twice daily, given to six patients normalized their thiamine status and improved left ventricular ejection fraction (LVEF) in four of five patients studied by echocardiography.

A more recent study by Shimon et al. found that thiamine repletion could improve left ventricular function and biochemical evidence of thiamine deficiency in some patients with moderate to severe CHF who were on long-term furosemide therapy (80 mg/day or more for at least 3 months).[2] In this double-blind, placebo-controlled trial, 30 patients were randomized to 1 week of inpatient therapy with either IV thiamine, 200 mg/day, or placebo. Following discharge, all 30 patients received oral thiamine, 200 mg/day for 6 weeks. After IV thiamine, the status of the vitamin normalized and LVEF significantly increased, compared to no changes with IV placebo. In the 27 patients completing the full 7-week intervention, LVEF increased by 22%. These findings suggest that thiamine supplementation corrected a subclinical thiamine deficiency state and may be beneficial for some CHF patients taking furosemide.

Another trial suggests that loop diuretics may not be at fault in the observed thiamine deficiency in CHF patients and that inadequate dietary intake of thiamine may play a role.[3] In this study, 38 patients with CHF taking loop diuretics were examined; 10 were determined to be at risk for dietary thiamine inadequacy and 8 were determined to be thiamine deficient. Of those latter eight patients, only four achieved two thirds of the recommended daily intake, based on estimated thiamine intake from a food frequency questionnaire. The authors note that individuals with CHF may have poor nutriture due to illness-related loss of appetite or age. Additionally, dietary sodium restrictions may remove from the menu many foods that would ordinarily contribute dietary thiamine.

Regardless of the explanation for deficiency, thiamine supplementation may be warranted.

Management Suggestions

Thiamine supplementation may prevent or correct thiamine deficiency and improve cardiac function in patients with CHF.

VITAMIN B₂ (RIBOFLAVIN)— ORAL CONTRACEPTIVES

Rating 3

Interaction Summary

Oral contraceptives (OCs) may deplete vitamin B_2 to some degree.

Discussion

Numerous studies indicate that OC use may impair vitamin B_2 status, especially in those taking OCs for a long period of time.[1-3] Under ordinary circumstances, however, OC use appears unlikely to produce clinical effects of vitamin B_2 deficiency.

Management Suggestions

Though OC use is unlikely to produce clinical effects of vitamin B_2 deficiency under ordinary circumstances, B_2 supplementation at standard nutritional doses may be advisable on general principles for women using OCs.

Rating Scale:
(1) Significant interaction
(2) Possibly significant interaction

(3) Interaction of relatively little significance
(4) Reported interaction that does not, in fact, exist or is insignificant

VITAMIN B$_6$ (PYRIDOXINE)—ISONIAZID

Rating 1

RELATED DRUGS

Hydralazine
Isocarboxazid

Phenelzine

Interaction Summary

Isoniazid interferes with pyridoxine activity. This effect appears to be dose related and can lead to the development of peripheral neuritis caused by pyridoxine deficiency. A possible complicating factor is that excessive supplemental pyridoxine may blunt the therapeutic effects of isoniazid. Hydralazine, phenelzine, and isocarboxazid are structurally similar and may affect pyridoxine similarly.

Discussion

Isoniazid is a hydrazine that forms a hydrazone with pyridoxal-5-phosphate (the active form of pyridoxine), inhibiting its coenzyme action.[1,2]

Isoniazid-induced pyridoxine interference is dose related and leads to the development of peripheral neuritis with symptoms such as tingling and numbness of the fingers and toes. The con-

---

Rating Scale:
(1) Significant interaction
(2) Possibly significant interaction

(3) Interaction of relatively little significance
(4) Reported interaction that does not, in fact, exist or is insignificant

dition has been reported to occur in 44% of patients taking iso-niazid, 16 to 24 mg/kg/day, but in only 2% of patients taking 3 to 5 mg/kg/day.[3] However, even low doses of isoniazid (4 to 6 mg/kg/day) can produce a high incidence of neuropathy in mal-nourished patients and others predisposed to it, including preg-nant women, the elderly, diabetics, alcoholics, uremics, those with liver disease, and those who do not metabolize isoniazid properly.[4] The condition can be reversed by stopping the drug and administering supplemental B$_6$ in high doses (e.g., 100 to 200 mg/day).[3] For prevention of drug-induced peripheral neuropa-thy, smaller doses of B$_6$ (e.g., 6 to 50 mg/day) have been used.

The MAO inhibitor phenelzine is structurally similar, and there is a case report of pyridoxine-related peripheral neuropathy as-sociated with it.[2] The MAO inhibitor isocarboxazid, as well as the antihypertensive hydralazine, may also be implicated.

It may be advisable to keep pyridoxine doses low because high doses of the vitamin may interfere with isoniazid's antibacterial activity[3] and hydralazine's antihypertensive effect.[5]

Management Suggestions

Consider administering pyridoxine (6 to 50 mg/day) with iso-niazid to prevent drug-induced peripheral neuropathy. However, some clinicians recommend preventive pyridoxine therapy only for those predisposed to peripheral neuropathies, including pregnant women, the elderly, diabetics, alcoholics, uremics, those with liver disease, and those who don't metabolize isoni-azid properly.[4]

It should be noted that long-standing neuropathies caused by drug-induced pyridoxine deficiency may not respond to pyri-doxine repletion, so patients should be advised to report symp-toms as early as possible.[2]

VITAMIN B$_6$ (PYRIDOXINE)—LEVODOPA

Rating 3

Interaction Summary

Pyridoxine in larger doses can reduce the therapeutic effects of levodopa in Parkinson's disease.

Discussion

The recommended daily intake for pyridoxine in adults is 2 mg for men and 1.6 mg for women. Pyridoxine in higher doses of 5 to 25 mg has been reported to reduce the therapeutic effects of levodopa.

Conversion of dopa to dopamine in the brain is the basis for using levodopa (L-dopa) in Parkinson's disease. Pyridoxine appears to accelerate the peripheral metabolism of levodopa to dopamine and degradation products, leaving less levodopa available for conversion to dopamine in the brain. (Dopamine in the peripheral circulation does not cross the blood-brain barrier.) In one study, pyridoxine, 50 mg/day, was associated with a 66% reduction in plasma L-dopa levels and clinical deterioration of Parkinson's disease in three of four patients.[1] Because this interaction appears to occur only with larger pyridoxine doses, recommendation of a pyridoxine-deficient diet in patients taking levodopa is probably unnecessary[2] and could lead to a pyridoxine deficiency with its own adverse effects.

Rating Scale:
(1) Significant interaction
(2) Possibly significant interaction

(3) Interaction of relatively little significance
(4) Reported interaction that does not, in fact, exist or is insignificant

Carbidopa, which is usually given with levodopa, has the opposite effect of pyridoxine and generally neutralizes the vitamin's effect on levodopa. However, this neutralizing effect may depend to some degree on the doses of carbidopa and pyridoxine.

Management Suggestions

Avoid higher doses of pyridoxine supplements in individuals taking levodopa without carbidopa.

VITAMIN B$_6$ (PYRIDOXINE)— ORAL CONTRACEPTIVES

Rating 4

Interaction Summary

Although it is sometimes reported that oral contraceptives (OCs) may adversely affect vitamin B$_6$ status, more recent studies have not found such an effect.

Discussion

In a 1984 study, 115 women were administered a combination OC (levonorgestrel 150 μg/ethinyl estradiol 30 μg) and multivitamin supplement or placebo, while 19 women wearing an intrauterine contraceptive device (IUCD) and taking placebo served as controls.[1] Assessments were made at baseline and through 13 cycles of OC use. No significant adverse effects of the OC on vitamin B$_6$ status were found. Similarly, a 1989 6-month study in which 55 women were administered various brands of low-dose OCs found no adverse effects on B$_6$ status.[2]

A 1995 study of 14 young women administered a triphasic low-dose OC, and nine matched control subjects, found that short-term OC use (6 cycles) did not alter vitamin B$_6$ levels (as reflected by pyridoxal-5-phosphate, the active form of the vitamin) in plasma and erythrocytes in the majority of women consuming adequate diets.[3]

Rating Scale:
(1) Significant interaction
(2) Possibly significant interaction

(3) Interaction of relatively little significance
(4) Reported interaction that does not, in fact, exist or is insignificant

Management Suggestions

Although OCs do not appear to affect vitamin B$_6$ status, B$_6$ deficiency is relatively common.[4-6] For this reason, vitamin B$_6$ supplementation at standard nutritional doses may be appropriate on general principles.

VITAMIN B$_6$ (PYRIDOXINE)— PENICILLAMINE

Rating 3

Interaction Summary

Indirect evidence suggests that penicillamine therapy could possibly induce pyridoxine deficiency.

Discussion

Penicillamine might lead to pyridoxine deficiency, according to tests on blood samples drawn from rheumatoid arthritis (RA) patients receiving various dosages of the drug.[1] Serving as controls were RA patients taking antiinflammatory agents other than penicillamine, drugs considered unlikely to affect vitamin B$_6$ status, or no medication.

Vitamin B$_6$ deficiency was assessed in vitro by measuring the percentage stimulation of erythrocyte alanine aminotransferase (ALT) when an excess of pyridoxal-5-phosphate (PLP) was added to the blood sample. (This technique is an alternative to the more common method of assessing penicillamine-induced pyridoxine deficiency by measuring urinary xanthurenic acid excretion following an oral tryptophan load test.) Because ALT is a PLP-dependent apoenzyme, PLP-depleted ALT (caused by penicillamine) will replenish itself by taking up available PLP and thus become more active. The unstimulated ALT activity of penicillamine-treated subjects was significantly lower than that

---

Rating Scale:
(1) Significant interaction
(2) Possibly significant interaction

(3) Interaction of relatively little significance
(4) Reported interaction that does not, in fact, exist or is insignificant

274

of controls, as would be expected if ALT were deficient in its PLP coenzyme.

Compared to controls, in vitro ALT stimulation by PLP was less marked at intermediate penicillamine dosage levels. This possibly suggests that a pyridoxine deficiency may occur in the early stage of treatment with penicillamine and that some recovery then takes place, with the deficiency recurring only in cases in which the penicillamine dose is subsequently raised to a high level. However, there were no clinical signs of pyridoxine deficiency, so pyridoxine supplementation would appear unnecessary except in those patients with poor nutritional status.

Management Suggestions

Although penicillamine appears to deplete pyridoxine, this effect may be clinically important only in patients with poor nutritional status. However, because vitamin B$_6$ deficiency is relatively common,[2-4] supplementation in standard nutritional doses may be advisable on general principles.

VITAMIN B$_6$ (PYRIDOXINE)— THEOPHYLLINE

Rating 3

RELATED DRUGS

Aminophylline   Oxtriphylline
Dyphylline

Interaction Summary

Long-term theophylline treatment may deplete body stores of pyridoxine and pyridoxine supplementation may restore normal pyridoxine status. Very preliminary evidence suggests that pyridoxine supplementation may also reduce adverse nervous system effects, such as hand tremor, associated with theophylline use.

Discussion

Pyridoxal kinase metabolizes pyridoxine to its active form, pyridoxal-5-phosphate (PLP). Theophylline is a pyridoxine antagonist, apparently due to its potent inhibition of pyridoxal kinase (PK).[1]

A study in 26 asthmatic children found a significant negative correlation between serum levels of PLP and theophylline in the 20 patients treated with slow-release theophylline compared to

Rating Scale:
(1) Significant interaction
(2) Possibly significant interaction

(3) Interaction of relatively little significance
(4) Reported interaction that does not, in fact, exist or is insignificant

the six patients receiving no theophylline (mean ± SEM): 5.3 ± 0.5 versus 9.0 ± 1.4 ng/ml; $P < 0.05$.[2] Circulating PLP levels fell quickly, just after theophylline treatment was started. All the patients consumed the same diet and were almost identical in nutritional status.

Another study found a similar rapid and significant decline in both plasma and erythrocyte PLP levels. This 16-week trial involving seven healthy male volunteers examined the effect of long-term theophylline treatment on pyridoxine homeostasis.[3] Mean erythrocyte ALT and AST enzyme activity declined by 70% and 50%, respectively, indicating that decreased availability of PLP can have widespread metabolic consequences. The observed threefold increase in total erythrocyte PK activity levels may have been a compensatory attempt to raise PLP levels, but this did not normalize either plasma or erythrocyte PLP levels. This suggests that theophylline's effect on pyridoxine metabolism is not transitory and cannot be overcome by elevated intracellular levels of PK. However, supplementation with pyridoxine HCl 10 mg/day for 1 week normalized indices of pyridoxine status and reversed the downward trend in both ALT and AST activity levels.

A 6-week, placebo-controlled crossover study in 15 healthy volunteers found that plasma PLP levels significantly declined in those taking a combination of slow-release theophylline (5 to 8 mg/kg/day) and pyridoxal HCl (15 mg/day). Even so, PLP levels remained above the normal reference range (30 to 80 nM/L) during the study period, indicating that functional pyridoxine status was more than adequate.[1]

These findings suggest that theophylline-induced pyridoxine deficiency can be prevented by pyridoxine supplementation.

There is also evidence that pyridoxine supplementation may reduce some theophylline-related adverse effects. A randomized double-blind, placebo-controlled crossover study involving 20 healthy young healthy adults found that theophylline-related hand tremor after a single dose of the drug was markedly reduced ($P < 0.01$) with pyridoxine supplementation (pyridoxal HCl 15 mg/day), and a similar but not statistically significant trend was observed with repeated drug doses.[4] Pyridoxine supplementation also appeared to reduce many other side effects related to nervous system function (particularly feeling faint, trembling, and irritability), suggesting that theophylline-related adverse effects may be at least partly due to the drug's effect on pyridoxine.

One explanation for reduced tremor may be a modulating effect by pyridoxine on catecholamine release, which has been associated with both pyridoxine deficiency (in rats)[5] and theophylline therapy.[6] The differences observed between single and repeated doses of theophylline might be explained by adaptation to theophylline or by deterioration in pyridoxine status. A higher pyridoxine dose may be needed to sustain a significant reduction in theophylline-induced hand tremor.

Management Suggestions

Pyridoxine supplementation may be advisable during long-term theophylline treatment. Pyridoxine 10 to 15 mg/day may help maintain normal pyridoxine status. Higher doses may reduce theophylline-related hand tremor and other adverse effects, but this has not been established.

VITAMIN B$_{12}$—COLCHICINE

Rating 3

Interaction Summary

Chronic use of colchicine can impair intestinal absorption of vitamin B$_{12}$.

Discussion

Absorption studies using the Schilling test in 20 participants taking oral colchicine found significantly reduced vitamin B$_{12}$ absorption in all but one subject.[1] No effect on intrinsic factor was observed; the most likely mechanism is colchicine's effect on the ileal site of vitamin B$_{12}$ absorption.

Management Suggestions

Serum B$_{12}$ measurement and supplementation as needed may be warranted during extended colchicine therapy.

Rating Scale:
(1) Significant interaction
(2) Possibly significant interaction

(3) Interaction of relatively little significance
(4) Reported interaction that does not, in fact, exist or is insignificant

VITAMIN B$_{12}$—H$_2$ ANTAGONISTS

Rating 2

RELATED DRUGS

Cimetidine	Nizatidine
Famotidine	Omeprazole
Lansoprazole	Ranitidine

Interaction Summary

H$_2$ antagonists and other drugs that inhibit gastric acid secretion may reduce the absorption of vitamin B$_{12}$ from foods. However, the absorption of oral B$_{12}$ supplements should not be affected.

Discussion

Adequate stomach acid and pepsin are required to free cobalamin (vitamin B$_{12}$) from its dietary protein-bound form. Vitamin B$_{12}$ is then attached to intrinsic factor, which allows the vitamin to be absorbed in the intestines. The H$_2$ antagonist cimetidine given four times daily (1000 mg total) reduced the absorption of dietary vitamin B$_{12}$ in both peptic ulcer patients and normal subjects, compared to baseline, confirming findings in other studies.[1] However, 400 mg of cimetidine given at night had no significant effect on dietary vitamin B$_{12}$ absorption.

The latter finding may be explained by the fact that the single night dose of cimetidine was given several hours after the last

Rating Scale:

(1) Significant interaction

(2) Possibly significant interaction

(3) Interaction of relatively little significance

(4) Reported interaction that does not, in fact, exist or is insignificant

meal of the day and so had little or no effect on vitamin B$_{12}$ absorption from that meal. However, when cimetidine is given in divided doses during the day, malabsorption of dietary vitamin B$_{12}$ is likely to occur. Long-term treatment could result in a vitamin B$_{12}$ deficiency, especially if body stores of B$_{12}$ are already low.

In another study, 13 peptic ulcer patients given cimetidine, 300 mg, 30 minutes before eating eggs containing radiolabeled vitamin B$_{12}$ experienced a significant decreased absorption (53%) of the labeled B$_{12}$.[2] However, cimetidine had no significant effect on the absorption of supplemental oral crystalline vitamin B$_{12}$. Another histamine H$_2$ antagonist, ranitidine, also has been found to cause malabsorption of dietary vitamin B$_{12}$.[3]

Studies of the proton pump inhibitor omeprazole produced similar findings. The effect of omeprazole on dietary vitamin B$_{12}$ was studied in seniors—eight taking omeprazole, eight normal subjects, and three with atrophic gastritis.[4] Omeprazole treatment and atrophic gastritis both decreased dietary B$_{12}$ absorption compared to the normal control group. Ingestion of cranberry juice or dilute HCl increased the absorption of dietary vitamin B$_{12}$ in both omeprazole-treated and atrophic gastritis patients.

Another study of 10 healthy males found that omeprazole therapy markedly decreased dietary vitamin B$_{12}$ absorption in a dose-dependent manner.[5] After 2 weeks, vitamin B$_{12}$ absorption decreased by 72% in those taking 20 mg of omeprazole daily and by 88% in those taking 40 mg daily.

Management Suggestions

Vitamin B$_{12}$ supplementation may be advisable to compensate for the malabsorption of dietary B$_{12}$ associated with H$_2$ antagonist or proton pump inhibitor therapy. However, single-dose therapy of H$_2$ blockers at night is unlikely to affect dietary B$_{12}$ absorption.

VITAMIN B$_{12}$—METFORMIN

Rating 3

RELATED DRUGS

Phenformin

Interaction Summary

The biguanide oral hypoglycemic drugs metformin and phenformin may cause malabsorption of vitamin B$_{12}$.

Discussion

The biguanide oral hypoglycemic drugs metformin and phenformin are known to be associated with malabsorption of vitamin B$_{12}$. Of 46 randomly selected diabetic patients on biguanide therapy, 30% were found to have malabsorption of vitamin B$_{12}$.[1] However, there is no evidence as yet of severe B$_{12}$ deficiency caused by these medications.

Interestingly, withdrawal from the drug resulted in normal vitamin B$_{12}$ absorption in only half of those with malabsorption while on biguanide therapy. This suggests that biguanides can induce B$_{12}$ malabsorption two different ways: one which is temporary and unrelated to intrinsic factor secretion and another which is permanent and mediated by the depression of intrinsic factor secretion. For this reason, it is unwise to assume that mal-

Rating Scale:
(1) Significant interaction
(2) Possibly significant interaction

(3) Interaction of relatively little significance
(4) Reported interaction that does not, in fact, exist or is insignificant

absorption of vitamin B$_{12}$ during biguanide therapy will invariably remit on drug withdrawal.

A recent comparative study involving patients with type 2 diabetes suggests that increased calcium intake may help correct this problem.[2] Of 21 participants on sulfonylurea therapy, 14 were switched to metformin and the remaining seven served as controls. The patients receiving metformin (up to 850 mg three times daily) were found to have diminished B$_{12}$ absorption and low serum total B$_{12}$ and holotranscobalamin II (holoTCII), the bioavailable form of B$_{12}$. After 3 months of metformin therapy, oral calcium carbonate (1.2 g/day) administered for 1 month partially reversed the effects of metformin on B$_{12}$. Mean serum holoTCII (baseline = 175 $\pm$ 19 pg/ml) increased by 53 $\pm$ 15% from month 3 to month 4 (111 $\pm$ 21 to 153 $\pm$ 11 pg/ml; $P < 0.005$). Serum total B$_{12}$ did not change significantly, but continued depression of holoTCII levels would be expected to be followed by low serum total B$_{12}$ levels and, presumably, eventual clinical B$_{12}$ deficiency. Based on findings from earlier studies,[3,4] it is believed that metformin interferes with calcium-dependent intestinal absorption of vitamin B$_{12}$.

Management Suggestions

This interaction is of particular concern because the peripheral neuropathy associated with diabetes may be indistinguishable from that associated with vitamin B$_{12}$ deficiency. It is advisable to monitor serum vitamin B$_{12}$ levels in patients taking metformin or phenformin. Keep in mind that discontinuation of the drug may not restore normal B$_{12}$ absorption. Based on recent evidence, increased calcium intake may be advisable to help prevent biguanide-induced B$_{12}$ malabsorption.

VITAMIN B$_{12}$—NITROUS OXIDE

Rating 1

OTHER POTENTIALLY IMPLICATED SUPPLEMENTS
Folate (folic acid)

Interaction Summary

Nitrous oxide can inactivate vitamin B$_{12}$ and cause neurologic deterioration in patients with existing vitamin B$_{12}$ deficiency. Secondary folate deficiency may also develop.

Discussion

Abundant evidence suggests that nitrous oxide inactivates vitamin B$_{12}$.[1,2] Active vitamin B$_{12}$ contains cobalt in its reduced form (Co^{1+}). Nitrous oxide irreversibly oxidizes reduced cobalt to the Co^{2+} and Co^{3+} forms, and renders vitamin B$_{12}$ inactive. This in turn reduces the activity of the cobalamin-dependent enzyme methionine synthetase, resulting in decreased production of methionine as well as tetrahydrofolate, which is required in DNA synthesis.[3]

Inactivated vitamin B$_{12}$ is normally rapidly replaced, but not in individuals with existing B$_{12}$ deficiency. For this reason, short-term exposure to nitrous oxide in healthy individuals appears to cause no significant problems. However, long-term exposure can produce megaloblastic anemia and neurologic changes.

Rating Scale:
(1) Significant interaction
(2) Possibly significant interaction

(3) Interaction of relatively little significance
(4) Reported interaction that does not, in fact, exist or is insignificant

One report reviewed four prior cases and one present case in which patients with unsuspected vitamin B$_{12}$ deficiency developed subacute combined degeneration of the spinal cord following nitrous oxide anesthesia.[2] The findings suggested that patients with B$_{12}$ deficiency are especially sensitive to neurologic deterioration following nitrous oxide anesthesia. If unrecognized, this neurologic deterioration can become irreversible and result in death.

A study compared 40 patients before and after surgery under nitrous oxide anesthesia to 12 control subjects anesthetized with total intravenous anesthesia. Cobalamin-dependent methionine synthesis was found to become seriously compromised during nitrous oxide anesthesia, leading to elevated plasma homocysteine levels, which may therefore be used for monitoring nitrous oxide–induced cobalamin inactivation.[4] Disturbances of homocysteine and folate metabolism by nitrous oxide develop quickly, and a return to normal levels requires several days.

A study of 48 patients admitted to an intensive care unit and given nitrous oxide anesthesia found that secondary development of folate deficiency from nitrous oxide–induced effects may occur in some seriously ill patients and in turn may result in the persistence and possible progression of bone marrow abnormalities.[1] For this reason, consideration should be given to early supplementation with folic acid in such patients.

In a previous study of 70 seriously ill patients admitted to an ICU, no evidence of folate deficiency was found in those who had not received nitrous oxide, but evidence of a disturbance in folate metabolism was present in a large proportion of those exposed to nitrous oxide anesthesia.[3] The development of megaloblastic changes in ICU patients may depend on other factors related to the acute illness in addition to nitrous oxide anesthesia.

However, nitrous oxide–induced disturbances in vitamin B$_{12}$ and folate metabolism may not necessarily be clinically important.[5] Of 49 patients exposed to isoflurane alone or combined with nitrous oxide, a small, transient disruption in folate metabolism (based on an increase in the formiminoglutamic acid/creatinine ratio) occurred in those undergoing acoustic neuroma resection and given nitrous oxide (mean anesthesia duration of 9.3 hours) but not in those having hip replacement surgery. This effect peaked at the end of anesthetic exposure and returned toward control levels by the first day after anesthesia and surgery, and would not be expected to have clinical consequences. Low preoperative levels of red blood cell folate and low-normal levels of serum vitamin B$_{12}$ were not predictive of this response to nitrous oxide.

Folinic acid (leucovorin) appears to offset the effect of nitrous oxide and rapidly restore a normal marrow, and in one case report has been found to be effective following nitrous oxide exposure lasting 24 hours.[6]

Management Suggestions

To avoid possible neurologic problems, anesthesiologists should avoid using nitrous oxide anesthesia in patients with vitamin B$_{12}$ deficiency.[2] Preoperative vitamin B$_{12}$ levels should be obtained in patients who have increased mean corpuscular volume indexes or previous gastric or intestinal resections so that a B$_{12}$ deficiency can be treated before and after surgery and anesthesia. If seriously ill individuals are given nitrous oxide, both vitamin B$_{12}$ and folate (or folinic acid) supplementation should be considered.

Professionals regularly exposed to nitrous oxide, such as dentists and dental hygienists, may be at risk for deficiency as well.

VITAMIN B$_{12}$—
ORAL CONTRACEPTIVES

Rating 4

Interaction Summary

Studies have found that women taking oral contraceptives (OCs) frequently have lower serum vitamin B$_{12}$ levels than women not using them. However, total vitamin B$_{12}$ stores apparently remain normal in OC users, and a B$_{12}$ deficiency may be unlikely to occur.

Discussion

A 1993 study examined the effects of oral folate loading in 29 long-term users of OCs containing less than 50 μg estrogen and 13 women serving as controls.[1] OC use decreased serum vitamin B$_{12}$ levels but did not significantly change B$_{12}$ status. An observational study of 229 adolescent females taking OCs also found decreased serum vitamin B$_{12}$ levels.[2]

However, in another observational study of 101 women taking OCs and 113 non-OC users serving as controls, evidence suggested that the lower serum vitamin B$_{12}$ levels observed in OC users were caused by decreased serum unsaturated B$_{12}$ binding capacity rather than by actual B$_{12}$ depletion.[3] Since none of the OC users had dietary vitamin B$_{12}$ insufficiency, findings of normal B$_{12}$ absorption and excretion indicated that their cobalamin stores were apparently normal. However, serum unsaturated B$_{12}$

Rating Scale:

(1) Significant interaction

(2) Possibly significant interaction

(3) Interaction of relatively little significance

(4) Reported interaction that does not, in fact, exist or is insignificant

binding capacity (S-UBBC) was decreased compared to controls. S-UBBC consists of two transport proteins, TC-I and TC-II. Cobalamin is bound primarily to TC-I; a decrease in this protein does not lead to clinical cobalamin deficiency, but can produce a "false low" serum cobalamin, which appears to be the most likely explanation for the lower serum B_{12} levels found.

Management Suggestions

Under ordinary circumstances, vitamin B_{12} supplementation may not be necessary in OC users.

VITAMIN C—ASPIRIN

Interaction Summary

Aspirin may deplete body stores of vitamin C, possibly leading to subclinical scurvy and increasing the risk of abnormal bleeding episodes.

Discussion

Aspirin is known to deplete tissue levels of vitamin C, and the low vitamin C levels seen in patients with rheumatoid arthritis have been attributed to aspirin therapy.

Though some reports have suggested otherwise, a study in guinea pigs suggests that aspirin apparently does not inhibit the absorption of vitamin C.[1] Rather, an in vitro study using bovine tissue indicates that aspirin competes with vitamin C for binding to plasma proteins and displaces vitamin C from these proteins.[2] This may be the primary mechanism for the interaction. The result would be reduced body stores of protein-bound vitamin C and a temporary increase in free plasma vitamin C, which would then be rapidly metabolized or excreted. In this way, aspirin-induced vitamin C depletion could lead to the onset of subclinical scurvy.

Blood platelets appear to need vitamin C to clot normally.[3] Low vitamin C levels could enhance aspirin's anticoagulant effect and

Rating Scale:
(1) Significant interaction
(2) Possibly significant interaction

(3) Interaction of relatively little significance
(4) Reported interaction that does not, in fact, exist or is insignificant

increase the risk of hematemesis and other abnormal bleeding episodes.

Management Suggestions

Supplementary vitamin C may be beneficial during chronic aspirin therapy.

VITAMIN C—
ORAL CONTRACEPTIVES

Rating 3

Interaction Summary

Oral contraceptives (OCs) may depress blood levels of vitamin C.

Discussion

In a 1972 study, researchers controlled vitamin C intake over two and a half menstrual cycles in six young women: four of the women took OCs and two served as control subjects.[1] Fasting plasma vitamin C concentrations were determined to be saturated for each subject at the 150-mg/day controlled dietary intake. Vitamin C levels were measured at intervals, including during menses when OC users were off the OC. Compared to controls, those taking OCs had lower plasma vitamin C concentrations. The findings suggest that OCs depress plasma vitamin C levels and prevent the sharp increase in these levels ordinarily associated with ovulation. Reduced vitamin C levels in OC users have also been reported in numerous other studies.[2-5]

However, these are all older studies, and it isn't clear whether today's low-estrogen OCs would produce the same effect.

Management Suggestions

Vitamin C supplementation in at least standard nutritional doses may be advisable in patients taking OCs.

Rating Scale:
(1) Significant interaction
(2) Possibly significant interaction
(3) Interaction of relatively little significance
(4) Reported interaction that does not, in fact, exist or is insignificant

VITAMIN D—CIMETIDINE

Interaction Summary

Cimetidine may interfere with vitamin D metabolism. Other H_2 antagonists may be unlikely to interact.

Discussion

Vitamin D is converted to its major circulating metabolite, 25-hydroxyvitamin D (25-OHD), by the hepatic microsomal enzyme vitamin D-25-hydroxylase. Cimetidine is known to inhibit several microsomal oxidase enzymes. If the drug inhibits vitamin D-25-hydroxylase, it would be expected to lower blood levels of 25-OHD.

To test this assumption, nine adults were given 400 mg of cimetidine twice daily for 4 weeks during the seasonal change from winter to summer, when days are becoming longer.[1] Though cimetidine did not lower the levels of 25-OHD, it did prevent the expected seasonal rise in these levels. Additionally, levels of 25-OHD increased significantly after cimetidine administration was stopped. These observations suggest that cimetidine treatment could potentially interfere with vitamin D metabolism, and confirms previous findings in animals.[2,3]

Management Suggestions

Vitamin D supplementation at standard nutritional levels might be warranted during long-term cimetidine therapy.

Rating Scale:
(1) Significant interaction
(2) Possibly significant interaction

(3) Interaction of relatively little significance
(4) Reported interaction that does not, in fact, exist or is insignificant

VITAMIN D—HEPARIN

Interaction Summary

High-dose or long-term use of heparin may interfere with the physiologic conversion of dietary vitamin D to its most active form. The result of this interference may be bone demineralization leading to osteoporosis. In pregnant women, heparin therapy has been associated with fractured and collapsed vertebrae.

Discussion

Heparin may interfere with conversion of the vitamin D metabolite 25-hydroxyvitamin D (25-OHD) to 1,25-dihydroxy-vitamin D or $1,25(OH)_2D$, the most active form of vitamin D.[1] Low blood levels of this active metabolite result in decreased calcium absorption. Additionally, heparin inhibits bone formation and promotes osteolysis, possibly by exerting a parathyroid hormone–like effect.[2] These effects combined may predispose individuals to osteoporosis. The results may be especially dramatic during pregnancy, with its increased calcium demand and decreased levels of calcitonin.

A 35-year-old woman who developed a deep vein thrombosis in her left leg early in pregnancy was treated with 30,000 IU heparin daily for 6 days and then 5000 IU three times daily for the rest of her pregnancy and afterward, for a total of 34 weeks.[2] She began suffering back pain during the last 2 weeks of pregnancy,

---

Rating Scale:
(1) Significant interaction
(2) Possibly significant interaction

(3) Interaction of relatively little significance
(4) Reported interaction that does not, in fact, exist or is insignificant

and 6 weeks after giving birth was diagnosed with a compression fracture of a thoracic vertebra and appeared to have osteoporosis in the spinal column. She had no identifiable risks for osteoporosis other than heparin use. Her levels of the active vitamin D metabolite $1,25(OH)_2D$ were well below normal during heparin treatment and returned to normal after heparin was discontinued.

Another pregnant woman sustained multiple vertebral compression fractures during 9 months of heparin therapy for prevention of thromboembolism.[3] She self-administered heparin, 10,000 IU subcutaneously twice daily, which was reduced to 8000 IU twice daily after problems developed. Severe back pain led to the diagnosis of osteoporosis with collapse of a lumbar vertebra as well as compression fractures of several other vertebrae.

A controlled study of 10 pregnant women confirmed that heparin therapy was associated with significantly lower levels of active vitamin D.[1] The treatment group received routine preventive heparin therapy at a dose of 5000 IU three times daily, and both treatment and control groups were given 400 IU of a vitamin D supplement daily. This interaction may be of clinical importance only in patients taking long-term high-dose heparin therapy, and the lower doses used in thromboembolism prevention do not appear to significantly impair the production of active vitamin D. However, it must be noted that heparin-treated patients took supplementary vitamin D, which could have limited the fall in their active vitamin D levels.

Management Suggestions

Supplementary vitamin D and calcium might be expected to help prevent heparin-induced osteoporosis. Monitoring of bone density during long-term heparin therapy might also be advisable.

VITAMIN D—ISONIAZID

Rating 3

Interaction Summary

The antituberculosis drug isoniazid may interfere with the activity of vitamin D, leading to decreased blood levels of calcium and phosphate. However, homeostatic mechanisms may make these effects clinically unimportant with long-term therapy. The same seems to be the case for combination antituberculosis therapy with isoniazid and rifampin.

Discussion

Isoniazid appears to inhibit the hepatic and renal hydroxylase enzymes needed to form two vitamin D metabolites: 1,25-dihydroxyvitamin D or $1,25(OH)_2D$, the most active vitamin D metabolite, and its precursor 25-hydroxyvitamin D (25-OHD), the major circulating metabolite.

A 14-day study in eight healthy men found that isoniazid, 300 mg/day, produced a consistent fall in serum levels of calcium and phosphate over the 2-week period, but that homeostatic mechanisms restored levels to normal.[1] After a single isoniazid dose, $1,25(OH)_2D$ levels fell by 47% and were reduced throughout the study. Levels of 25-OHD also declined, though much more slowly. However, the resultant relative hypocalcemia stimulated parathyroid hormone levels to rise by 36%; that response, combined with other homeostatic mechanisms, tended to bring

---

Rating Scale:
(1) Significant interaction
(2) Possibly significant interaction

(3) Interaction of relatively little significance
(4) Reported interaction that does not, in fact, exist or is insignificant

mineral blood levels back into balance, suggesting that the clinical effect of the interaction may be small.

Another homeostatic mechanism may help to explain findings that isoniazid does not seem to significantly affect calcium levels or bone development.[2] Low 25-OHD levels have been shown to step up activity of the renal enzyme that metabolizes 25-OHD to $1,25(OH)_2D$. In this way, normal $1,25(OH)_2D$ levels could be maintained despite lowered 25-OHD levels.

A 9-month study found that combination therapy with rifampin and isoniazid in eight tuberculosis patients appeared not to significantly alter vitamin D metabolism or calcium levels.[3] When viewed as a group, there were no significant changes from initial values for either the active metabolite $1,25(OH)_2D$ or its precursor 25-OHD. Radiocalcium absorption showed no significant changes after 3 months of treatment and there was little or no evidence of bone disease. Individuals more at risk appear to be those with increased calcium requirements (children and pregnant women) and Asians whose diets are often deficient in vitamin D, such as those in this study who had moved from India to Britain, where, additionally, the ultraviolet radiation is less.

Management Suggestions

Patients with already compromised calcium homeostasis or vitamin D nutriture should be carefully monitored while taking isoniazid alone or in combination with rifampin.

VITAMIN D—PHENYTOIN

RELATED DRUGS

Carbamazepine	Phenobarbital
Ethotoin	Primidone
Mephenytoin	Valproic acid

Interaction Summary

Phenytoin and other anticonvulsant drugs (including phenobarbital, primidone, and carbamazepine) that induce hepatic enzymes may interfere with vitamin D activity and thereby impair calcium utilization. Valproic acid may also be implicated through a different mechanism. This interference may increase the risk of osteoporosis and related bone disorders.

Discussion

Chronic therapy with phenytoin and other anticonvulsants is associated with bone-related problems such as rickets (in children) and osteomalacia (adult rickets). These agents are known to induce the hepatic metabolism of a number of drugs and appear likewise to induce the metabolic inactivation of vitamin D. They may also reduce calcium levels by direct effects on parathyroid hormone and calcium absorption.

Rating Scale:
(1) Significant interaction
(2) Possibly significant interaction
(3) Interaction of relatively little significance
(4) Reported interaction that does not, in fact, exist or is insignificant

Vitamin D is metabolized in the liver to 25-hydroxyvitamin D (25-OHD), which is further metabolized in the kidneys to 1,25-dihydroxyvitamin D or $1,25(OH)_2D$; this latter metabolite, the most active form of vitamin D, exists in much smaller concentrations than its precursor[1] and is the form that regulates calcium and phosphorus transport.[2]

In a survey of outpatients with epilepsy who were receiving chronic combination therapy with phenytoin and phenobarbital, Hahn et al. found significant hypocalcemia in 19% of the 48 patients and significantly decreased serum levels of 25-OHD in 33%, as compared to 38 untreated controls.[3] Serum calcium was significantly lower in treated patients than control (mean ± SEM): 9.33 ± 0.05 versus 9.78 ± 0.06 ng/ml; $P < 0.001$. Likewise, serum 25-OHD was significantly lower in treated patients than control: 12.8 ± 0.8 versus 20.5 ± 1.0 ng/ml; $P < 0.001$. Similar but less marked changes were observed in 13 patients on chronic monotherapy with either phenytoin or phenobarbital. The cause appears to be anticonvulsant-induced induction of hepatic 25-hydroxylation of both vitamin D and 25-OHD to inactive polar metabolites, resulting in decreased serum 25-OHD levels. The effect on serum levels seemed to be time dependent, because those patients on anticonvulsant therapy for 6 weeks or less had normal levels of calcium and vitamin D. For these reasons, patients on chronic anticonvulsant therapy, especially those on polytherapy and those with limited sunlight exposure, may benefit from vitamin D supplementation.

Numerous other studies have also found decreased plasma levels of 25-OHD in patients taking anticonvulsants. Jubiz et al. used a radio-receptor assay to test whether levels of the active metabolite $1,25(OH)_2D$ might be decreased as well.[2] As it turned out, the 25 patients taking anticonvulsants (phenytoin and/or phenobarbital) had normal or increased plasma levels of $1,25(OH)_2D$ compared to the control group of 17 patients not taking the drugs. One possible explanation for this finding involves a homeostatic mechanism by which low 25-OHD levels step up the activity of the renal enzyme that metabolizes 25-

OHD to $1,25(OH)_2D$, thereby maintaining normal $1,25(OH)_2D$ levels despite lowered 25-OHD levels.[1]

To test the assumption that adequate sunlight exposure may compensate for anticonvulsant-induced interference with vitamin D metabolism, Williams et al. studied 450 patients with epilepsy residing in a Florida facility for the mentally retarded and who were receiving anticonvulsant therapy consisting of phenytoin, phenobarbital, and primidone, singly or in combination, as well as others.[4] None of the patients had low serum levels of vitamin D, as reflected by levels of 25-OHD, or radiologic evidence of rickets or osteomalacia. Only 55 were identified as being at risk for osteomalacia, as indicated by at least one abnormality in serum levels of calcium, phosphorus, or alkaline phosphatase. These findings suggest that environments providing opportunity for adequate sun exposure and hence, increased vitamin D levels, may greatly decrease the incidence of anticonvulsant-induced bone disorders.

Interestingly, an experimental study using rabbit tissue found that phenytoin and valproic acid *inhibited* the activity of the hepatic enzyme system that metabolizes vitamin D to 25-OHD, which would lead to decreased serum levels of this metabolite. Whether these enzyme-inhibiting effects in animal tissue might have clinical relevance in humans is uncertain.[5]

Although an alteration in vitamin D metabolism is generally thought to account for the decreased calcium levels observed with anticonvulsant therapy, Weinstein et al. reported that anticonvulsant-induced hypocalcemia could occur independently of effects on vitamin D metabolism.[6] In 109 ambulatory adult epileptic patients receiving chronic anticonvulsant therapy, 48% had serum ionized calcium values below normal compared to a control group. Hypocalcemia and osteopenia occurred despite normal mean levels of serum 25-OHD and $1,25(OH)_2D$. Reduced calcium levels were associated with secondary hyperparathyroidism, an expected compensatory response; however, the lack of full compensation suggests anticonvulsant drug interference with parathyroid hormone. These findings indicate that anticonvulsant-induced hypocalcemia with decreased bone mineral content may occur in the presence of normal circulating vitamin D metabolites. This could potentially play a greater role in the development of bone disorders than effects on vitamin D.

Wahl et al. also found an effect on calcium independent of vitamin D, though in this case it involved calcium absorption.[7] This study, involving 12 patients on long-term anticonvulsant therapy and 12 untreated age-matched control subjects, indicated the occurrence of some degree of calcium malabsorption in the presence of normal serum 25-OHD concentrations. Fractional calcium absorption was lower ($P < 0.025$) in the treated group (30.8% $\pm$ 3.7%) compared to the control group (42.2% $\pm$ 3.5%). Levels of $1,25(OH)_2D$ were not measured in this study.

Management Suggestions

Disorders of mineral metabolism should be ruled out before starting anticonvulsant therapy. In many cases, adequate sun exposure may compensate for anticonvulsant-induced impairment of vitamin D activity. Otherwise, vitamin D supplementation may be warranted.

VITAMIN D—RIFAMPIN

Rating 3

Interaction Summary

The antituberculosis drug rifampin may interfere with the activity of vitamin D. This effect, however, may not be clinically significant in most cases.

Discussion

Rifampin appears to decrease levels of 25-hydroxyvitamin D (25-OHD), the major circulating vitamin D metabolite, by inducing its metabolism to inactive forms.[1] This metabolite is the precursor to 1,25-dihydroxyvitamin D or $1,25(OH)_2D$, the most active form of vitamin D.

A 2-week treatment with rifampin, 600 mg/day, in eight patients produced a fall in plasma 25-OHD levels of about 70% but no effect on levels of $1,25(OH)_2D$, parathyroid hormone, or calcitonin.[2] The lack of an effect on $1,25(OH)_2D$ may have a homeostatic explanation. Low 25-OHD levels have been shown to step up the activity of the renal enzyme that metabolizes 25-OHD to $1,25(OH)_2D$.[2] In this way, normal $1,25(OH)_2D$ levels could be maintained despite lowered 25-OHD levels. These findings indicate little likelihood of a clinically relevant effect of rifampin on vitamin D activity.

Rating Scale:
(1) Significant interaction
(2) Possibly significant interaction

(3) Interaction of relatively little significance
(4) Reported interaction that does not, in fact, exist or is insignificant

Management Suggestions

Patients with already compromised calcium homeostasis or vitamin D nutriture should be carefully monitored while taking rifampin alone or in combination with isoniazid (see the **Vitamin D—Isoniazid** article).

VITAMIN K—AMOXICILLIN

Rating 4

RELATED DRUGS

Fluoroquinolones   Sulfonamides
Macrolides   Tetracyclines
Penicillins

Interaction Summary

Although the evidence is weak, antibiotic treatment might impair vitamin K status in patients with existing low vitamin K levels. A potential interaction may be more consequential with certain cephalosporin antibiotics (see the **Vitamin K—Cephalosporins** article).

Discussion

It is widely believed that antibiotics can cause vitamin K deficiency by suppressing vitamin K–producing gut flora, but convincing evidence is lacking.[1] In a review, Lipsky found no definitive evidence that intestinal bacteria are an important nutritional source of vitamin K, and therefore, their suppression by broad-spectrum antibiotics might not even affect vitamin K levels.[2] However, there is at least some support for the idea.

Rating Scale:
(1) Significant interaction
(2) Possibly significant
     interaction

(3) Interaction of relatively little
     significance
(4) Reported interaction that
     does not, in fact, exist or is
     insignificant

An analysis of postmortem human liver samples appears to provide indirect evidence that the form of vitamin K produced by bacteria is absorbed from the distal intestinal tract and might play a significant role in meeting vitamin K requirements in the absence of dietary vitamin K.[3] Of the 22 deceased, 9 had been ill and were receiving broad-spectrum antimicrobials, and 13 were apparently healthy individuals who were victims of unexpected sudden death. No significant differences were found in average hepatic phylloquinone (dietary vitamin K) content between the two groups; however, there was a significant reduction in total hepatic menaquinone (bacteria-produced vitamin K) content in the antibiotic-treated group compared to the other group.

If symptomatic vitamin K deficiency due to the effects of antibiotics on gut flora does occur, it is probably limited to those individuals with preexisting low vitamin K levels.[1] In any case, patients with adequate nutritional status maintain normal prothrombin times regardless of the antibiotic administered.[1,4,5]

Management Suggestions

It may be advisable to give supplemental vitamin K, or to monitor prothrombin times, in patients with low vitamin K stores (caused by malnutrition, malabsorption, or total parenteral nutrition) who are treated with an antibiotic, particularly a cephalosporin containing the methyltetrazolethiol side chain (see the **Vitamin K—Cephalosporins** article).

VITAMIN K—CEPHALOSPORINS

Rating 3

RELATED DRUGS

Cefamandole	Ceftazidime
Cefazolin	Ceftizoxime
Cefonicid	Ceftriaxone
Cefoperazone	Cefuroxime
Cefotaxime	Cephalothin
Cefotetan	Cephapirin
Cefoxitin	Cephradine

Interaction Summary

Cephalosporins may impair vitamin K–dependent blood clotting in patients with vitamin K–poor diets, possibly leading to bleeding complications.

Discussion

Cephalosporins with a methyltetrazolethiol side chain (e.g., cefazolin, cefmetazole, cefoperazone, and cefotetan) may prolong prothrombin time, possibly leading to bleeding complications. The mechanism appears to be antibiotic-induced inhibition of the hepatic vitamin K–vitamin K epoxide cycle, probably by interference with vitamin K epoxide reductase activity, similar to the way anticoagulants such as warfarin work but to a lesser

Rating Scale:
(1) Significant interaction
(2) Possibly significant interaction
(3) Interaction of relatively little significance
(4) Reported interaction that does not, in fact, exist or is insignificant

extent.[1,2] This metabolic cycle produces the active vitamin K quinol form. Cephalosporin-induced inhibition of the cycle appears to be relatively weak, because a diet providing adequate vitamin K is usually enough to overcome it.

However, not all findings support the importance of the methyltetrazolethiol side chain in this potential interaction. An observational study of 546 critically ill patients suggested that this side chain alone may not be an independent risk factor for increased bleeding tendency.[3] Data from another human study indicate that methyltetrazolethiol side chain antibiotics may not affect blood clotting any more than other antibiotics, suggesting that the clotting impairment observed among patients receiving these antibiotics must be more complex and may be dependent on a number of unidentified factors.[4]

Shearer et al. investigated the effects of cephalosporin-induced hypoprothrombinemia in 49 hospitalized patients receiving antibiotics, with 67 untreated subjects serving as controls.[2] Prothrombin times for 30 patients eating ordinary diets (with vitamin K levels in the normal range of 176 to 1184 pg/ml) remained normal during treatment with all six side chain cephalosporins tested (latamoxef, cefmenoxime, cefoperazone, cefotetan, cefamandole, and cefazolin). This contrasted with findings in 19 parenterally fed patients, 7 of whom were treated with a cephalosporin antibiotic containing a methyltetrazolethiol side chain (latamoxef) and 12 with a cephalosporin without the side chain (cefotaxime or cefoxitin). All had lower plasma vitamin K levels (50 to 790 pg/ml) but normal clotting before starting antibiotic therapy. Only those patients treated with the side-chain antibiotic developed prolonged prothrombin times. One mg of vitamin K given IV readily reversed the antibiotic-induced clotting impairment, but it recurred within 2 to 3 days. These findings suggest that low nutritional vitamin K status predisposes to antibiotic-induced blood clotting impairment.

Another study similarly found no adverse clotting effects in nine well-nourished patients with normal serum vitamin K levels (mean 546, range 310 to 1350 pg/ml) who were treated with a side-chain cephalosporin (cefotetan IV) for 7 days.[1] Of 20 other patients (surgery patients with normal prothrombin times) given IV antibiotics, 13 were given cefotetan (side-chain cephalosporin), five were given cephradine (non–side-chain cephalosporin) combined with metronidazole, and two were given gentamicin, penicillin, and metronidazole. Eleven patients developed prolonged prothrombin times after 3 to 7 days of antibiotic therapy. Of these 11 patients, 9 had clinical evidence of malnutrition and 9 had subnormal serum vitamin K levels (mean 119, range 43 to 354 pg/ml) before antibiotic therapy. Altogether, eight of nine patients had low serum vitamin K coexistent with poor nutritional status, despite an initially normal PT, and this was associated with a high incidence of hypoprothrombinemia following the antibiotic therapy. The added stress of surgery with limited food intake for several days afterward further added to the risk of hypoprothrombinemia. Notably, 4 of the 11 patients who developed prolonged prothrombin times received a non–side-chain antibiotic or an antibiotic of a different class, suggesting that antibiotics other than side-chain cephalosporins may also act as weak inhibitors of the vitamin K epoxide cycle. These findings suggest a firm connection between malnutrition and antibiotic-induced blood-clotting impairment.

In an observational study of 546 critically ill patients selected (based on serum albumin levels) to represent a nutritionally deficient population, Goss et al. provided additional evidence that poor nutritional status (without vitamin K supplementation) may be the key factor in increasing the risk of bleeding and hypoprothrombinemia, regardless of antibiotic therapy.[3]

It is widely believed that antibiotics in general may cause vitamin K deficiency by suppressing vitamin K–producing gut flora, but convincing evidence is lacking.[1,3,5] (See the **Vitamin K—Amoxicillin** article.)

Management Suggestions

It may be advisable to give supplemental vitamin K, or to monitor prothrombin times, in patients with low vitamin K stores (caused by malnutrition, malabsorption, or total parenteral nutrition) who are treated with a cephalosporin, particularly one containing the methyltetrazolethiol side chain. This interaction may not be significant in well-nourished patients with normal plasma vitamin K levels.

VITAMIN K—PHENYTOIN

Rating 2

RELATED DRUGS

Carbamazepine   Phenobarbitol
Ethotoin   Primidone
Mephenytoin

Interaction Summary

Phenytoin and other anticonvulsants (phenobarbital, primidone, and carbamazepine) that induce hepatic enzymes may interfere with vitamin K activity and cause a vitamin K deficiency in infants born to mothers taking these drugs. This may result in bleeding disorders or facial bone abnormalities.

Discussion

By inducing microsomal oxidase enzymes, phenytoin increases the metabolic breakdown of vitamin K. This may in turn lead to vitamin K deficiency in neonates exposed to anticonvulsant drugs prenatally, according to two studies. One study involved 25 pregnant women receiving anticonvulsant therapy and 25 pregnant women serving as controls,[1] and the other was a case-control study of 16 pregnant women on anticonvulsant therapy.[2] Though the mothers taking anticonvulsants had decreased vitamin K plasma concentrations themselves, true vitamin K deficiency was not prevalent.

Rating Scale:

(1) Significant interaction
(2) Possibly significant interaction

(3) Interaction of relatively little significance
(4) Reported interaction that does not, in fact, exist or is insignificant

The chief concern is an increased risk of bleeding disorders in newborns caused by depression of vitamin K–dependent coagulation factors. Additionally, facial deformities (maxillonasal hypoplasia) have occurred in children born to women taking anticonvulsants; these deformities may result from the reduction in vitamin K–dependent proteins that are important for normal calcium metabolism in bone, although other explanations have also been proposed.[3]

Management Suggestions

In mothers taking enzyme-inductive anticonvulsant therapy, vitamin K supplementation may be warranted to prevent neonatal bleeding disorders and congenital facial abnormalities.

WARFARIN—COENZYME Q$_{10}$

RELATED DRUGS

Anisindione   Dicumarol

Interaction Summary

Coenzyme Q$_{10}$ (CoQ$_{10}$) may interfere with the anticoagulant effects of warfarin.

Discussion

CoQ$_{10}$ is chemically related to menaquinone (vitamin K$_2$) and may possess procoagulational effects. In rats, CoQ$_{10}$ antagonism has been shown to increase prothrombin time.[1] Conversely, CoQ$_{10}$ may have vitamin K–antagonist actions in vitro, but this effect has not been confirmed in vivo.[2]

In three case reports, patients experienced a decrease in INR after the addition of CoQ$_{10}$ to their warfarin regimen.[3] A 68-year-old man on warfarin and other medications for 6 years showed a decreased INR 2 weeks after starting CoQ$_{10}$, 30 mg/day. Stopping CoQ$_{10}$ and temporarily increasing the warfarin dose stabilized his INR. A 72-year-old man with a pulmonary embolism was initially treated with heparin and warfarin and then warfarin alone. Several weeks later, low INR values were observed. It was

---

Rating Scale:
(1) Significant interaction
(2) Possibly significant
     interaction

(3) Interaction of relatively little
     significance
(4) Reported interaction that
     does not, in fact, exist or is
     insignificant

discovered that the patient had taken CoQ_{10} for 3 months before the embolism and also had taken CoQ_{10} during the times his INR values were low. A 70-year-old woman on warfarin and other medications for several years experienced a sudden drop in her INR when she took CoQ_{10}, 30 mg/day, for 2 weeks. Stopping CoQ_{10} and temporarily increasing the warfarin dose returned her INR to normal.

Management Suggestions

Avoid this combination or carefully monitor coagulation parameters and adjust the warfarin dose as warranted.

WARFARIN—DANSHEN

Rating 1

RELATED DRUGS

Anisindione   Dicumarol

Interaction Summary

Case reports and animal studies suggest that patients previously stabilized on warfarin may experience a significant increase in their prothrombin times if danshen is added to their regimen. One case report suggests that a combination of the herbs boldo and fenugreek might have the same effect.

Discussion

Danshen, a Chinese folk medicine, is the root of *Salvia miltorrhiza*. In traditional Chinese medicine, it is used for treatment of coronary artery disease.

In three reported cases, severe overanticoagulation and bleeding complications developed when patients on chronic warfarin therapy started using danshen.[1]

A danshen preparation in a concentration of 2 g/ml was administered to 10 rats at a fixed dose of 5 g/kg intraperitoneally twice daily versus saline controls.[2] After 3 days of treatment, warfarin

---

Rating Scale:
(1) Significant interaction
(2) Possibly significant interaction
(3) Interaction of relatively little significance
(4) Reported interaction that does not, in fact, exist or is insignificant

was administered orally as a single dose (2 mg/kg). At 48 hours, the AUC for warfarin was 154.8 ± 72.3 µg × hr/ml versus 269.5 ± 90.8 µg × hr/ml with danshen ($P < 0.005$). The half-life of warfarin decreased from 31.8 ± 0.8 hr to 16.0 ± 2.6 hr with danshen ($P < 0.001$), and the C_{max} nearly doubled from 5500 ± 1626 to $10,976 \pm 3975$ ng/ml ($P < 0.001$). In this study, danshen was not found to have any independent effect on coagulation (no significant change in prothrombin time), but it did increase the PT in patients on warfarin from 41.1 ± 3.4 to 49.9 ± 4.2 seconds. The PT returned to normal within 3 days following discontinuation of danshen.

Further study is needed of the active components of danshen (e.g., tanshinone and isothanshinone).

Management Suggestions

Preliminary data suggest that danshen may increase the anticoagulant activity of warfarin.

Because warfarin is a drug with a narrow therapeutic window having little margin for error, it is recommended that clinicians advise their patients to avoid concomitant use until more definitive data are available.

WARFARIN—DONG QUAI

Rating 2

RELATED DRUGS

Anisindione   Dicumarol

OTHER POTENTIALLY IMPLICATED SUPPLEMENTS

Chamomile   Horse chestnut
Dandelion   Red clover

Interaction Summary

Dong quai may potentiate the anticoagulant activity of warfarin, possibly due to its phytocoumarin content. Other herbs with high levels of phytocoumarins, such as chamomile, dandelion, horse chestnut, and red clover, may present similar risks.

Discussion

Concurrent administration of dong quai (from the dried root of *Radix angelica sinensis*), 565 mg once to twice daily, with warfarin, 5 mg daily, resulted in a 2.5-fold increase in prothrombin times (PT) and INR in a previously stabilized patient.[1] This 46-year-old African-American woman had a past medical history of rheumatic heart disease, stroke, and atrial fibrillation for which she took warfarin, 5 mg daily, resulting in an INR between 2 and 3. With no other changes in medications, diet, or concurrent

Rating Scale:
(1) Significant interaction
(2) Possibly significant
     interaction

(3) Interaction of relatively little
     significance
(4) Reported interaction that
     does not, in fact, exist or is
     insignificant

conditions, her INR increased to 4.9 within 4 months of initiating dong quai. Within 4 weeks of discontinuing dong quai, her INR returned to the normal range (i.e., 2.48).

Supportive evidence for an interaction has also been found in studies of related species. Coumarins identified from the roots of *Angelica dahurica* include heptatriacontane, bergapten, beraptol, and nodakenin.[2] In a study in which 200 ml of an extemporaneously prepared 25% RAS solution was administered intravenously for 20 days, PT were significantly ($P < 0.0001$) longer in patients diagnosed with acute ischemic stroke ($n = 50$) than in control patients ($n = 46$), although specific PT values were not reported.[3] Furthermore, osthole, isolated from *Angelica pubescens*, has been shown to inhibit platelet thromboxane formation and phosphoinositides breakdown resulting in the inhibition of platelet aggregation.[4] At a concentration of 100 µg/ml, osthole caused complete inhibition of aggregation of arachidonic acid (100 µmol) and platelet activating factor (2 ng/ml) ($P < 0.001$).[4]

However, in a rabbit study, it did not appear that *Angelica sinensis* affected warfarin pharmacokinetics.[5] Daily subcutaneous warfarin doses (0.6 mg/kg) that had achieved steady state were followed by administration of daily oral *A. sinensis* doses (2 mg/kg administered twice daily) beginning on day 3. Warfarin pharmacokinetics including half-life, area under the curve, clearance, elimination rate constant, volume of distribution, maximum plasma warfarin concentration (C_{max}), and the time to achieve that concentration (T_{max}) were analyzed. None of these variables was affected by concurrent administration of *A. sinensis*.[5] Strangely, PT was actually found to be lowered.

More study is needed in humans with special attention to prothrombin times as well as platelet function.

Management Suggestions

Concurrent administration of warfarin and dong quai may result in disrupted anticoagulation control. The PT and bleeding times of these patients should be closely monitored.

WARFARIN—FEVERFEW

Rating 2

RELATED DRUGS

Abciximab

Alteplase

Anagrelide

Anisindione

Ardeparin

Aspirin

Cilostazol

Clopidogrel

Dalteparin

Danaparoid

Dicumarol

Dipyridamole

Enoxaparin

Eptifibatide

Heparin

Lepirudin

NSAIDs

Pentoxifylline

Reteplase

Streptokinase

Ticlodipine

Tirofiban

Urokinase

Interaction Summary

Feverfew might enhance the anticoagulant effect of warfarin.

Discussion

Feverfew inhibits platelet activity.[1,2] By neutralizing sulfhydryl groups, feverfew and one of its active components, parthenolide, inhibited the capacity of platelets to aggregate in an in vitro

---

Rating Scale:

(1) Significant interaction

(2) Possibly significant interaction

(3) Interaction of relatively little significance

(4) Reported interaction that does not, in fact, exist or is insignificant

study utilizing venous blood from healthy volunteers.[1] Makheja and Bailey concluded that feverfew antiplatelet effects were secondary to a phospholipase inhibitor preventing arachidonic acid release.[2]

In a study of rat peritoneal leukocytes and human polymorphonuclear leukocytes, leaves or infusions of feverfew irreversibly inhibited the generation of thromboxane B_2 and leukotriene B_4 in a dose-dependent manner.[3] In another study examining the effect of feverfew on platelets, both feverfew extract and parthenolide were effective inhibitors of [^{14}C] 5-HT secretion and aggregation induced by the phorbol ester PMA, ADP, arachidonic acid, collagen, the thromboxane mimetic U46619, the diacylglycerol analogue OAG, and epinephrine.[4]

Despite these findings, no clinical evidence exists that feverfew adversely affects platelet function. In a study of 10 patients who had taken feverfew for 3.5 to 8 years, platelet aggregation induced by ADP and thrombin was indistinguishable between the six patients taking feverfew and the four patients who had discontinued feverfew for 6 months.[5] Furthermore, warfarin's effect on coagulation is mediated through the clotting cascade, which is presumably not affected by feverfew. However, despite the differing underlying mechanisms, the effects might combine to increase bleeding risk if these agents are taken simultaneously.

Management Suggestions

Clinicians are advised to include feverfew in their list of herbs to inquire about if a patient previously stabilized on warfarin begins to experience symptoms associated with increased anticoagulation. It would be prudent to obtain a bleeding time to ascertain if platelet function has been adversely affected, especially if the INR/PT is within the normal range.

WARFARIN—GARLIC

RELATED DRUGS

Abciximab	Enoxaparin
Alteplase	Eptifibatide
Anagrelide	Heparin
Anisindione	Lepirudin
Ardeparin	NSAIDs
Aspirin	Pentoxifylline
Cilostazol	Reteplase
Clopidogrel	Streptokinase
Dalteparin	Ticlodipine
Danaparoid	Tirofiban
Dicumarol	Urokinase
Dipyridamole	

Interaction Summary

Garlic may potentiate the anticoagulant activity of warfarin and other drugs that affect hemostasis.

Discussion

The platelet-inhibiting effect of garlic has been demonstrated in a double-blind, placebo-controlled study in 60 volunteers.[1]

Rating Scale:
(1) Significant interaction
(2) Possibly significant interaction
(3) Interaction of relatively little significance
(4) Reported interaction that does not, in fact, exist or is insignificant

After 4 weeks of daily ingestion of 800 mg of powdered garlic (in coated tablets), the ratio of circulating platelet aggregates decreased by 10.3% ($P < 0.01$) and spontaneous platelet aggregation decreased by 56.3% ($P < 0.01$).[1]

An effect on platelets has also been found in a study of 34 patients administered 0.12 g/day of essential oil of garlic.[2] After 20 days of treatment, the maximum aggregation rate dropped from 30.37% to 21.21%, with an average decrease of $9.16 \pm 1.84\%$ ($P < 0.001$). In another study, this antiplatelet-aggregation effect was noted in six volunteers as early as 5 days after initiation of treatment.[3]

In order to understand the underlying mechanism of action, an aqueous extract of garlic was studied in blood collected from healthy volunteers.[4] It was found that garlic reduced the formation of thromboxane from exogenous arachidonate, inhibited the formation of thromboxane and lipooxygenase products formed in platelets preincubated with arachidonate, inhibited the phospholipase activity, and inhibited the incorporation of arachidonate into platelet phospholipids.[4] The uptake of calcium into platelets was inhibited, lowering cytosolic calcium concentrations. The authors therefore concluded the effect of garlic on platelets occurred at various stages of platelet aggregation.[4] Sharma and Nirmala found that garlic oil inhibited platelet adhesion on polycarbonate surfaces by approximately 50% (19.0 ± 1.4 platelet adhesion/mm^2 area with 0.0 mL garlic oil/ml of platelet-rich plasma [PRP] versus 11.0 ± 1.4 platelet adhesion/mm^2 area with 0.5 mL garlic oil/ml of PRP).[5] However, in another study, collagen-induced platelet aggregation was not influenced by dried garlic in 20 patients with hyperlipoproteinemia.[6]

Allicin, an active breakdown product of fresh garlic, has been shown to inhibit platelet aggregation.[7] Collagen-induced aggregation was reduced from 100% in controls to 0% with an aqueous extract of garlic.[7] Ajoene, another active component of garlic, has also been shown to inhibit platelet aggregation in a dose-dependent manner that synergistically potentiates the inhibition of aggregation by indomethacin and dipyridamole.[8] Furthermore, ajoene was found to inhibit prostaglandin synthetase (IC_{50} = 5.1 μM) and 5-lipoxygenase (IC_{50} = 1.6 μM) to approximately the same degree as that reported for indomethacin (IC_{50} = 0.8 μM).[9]

Garlic's influence on coagulation appears to have been the cause of platelet dysfunction with concomitant bleeding reported in an 87-year-old man.[10] This gentleman had self-administered approximately 2 g of garlic daily for an unspecified time period to prevent heart disease. He denied taking nonsteroidal antiinflammatory drugs, aspirin, or other medications known to alter hemostasis. He developed an unusual tendency to bruise easily followed by flaccid paralysis, loss of sensation below approximately T6, absent deep tendon reflex in the lower extremities, absent superficial abdominal and cremasteric reflexes, and loss of proprioception in both feet. His prothrombin time (PT) and partial thromboplastin time (PTT) were 12.7 and 22.3 seconds, respectively (control: 12 seconds). The platelet count was 178,000. A computed tomographic scan demonstrated a posterior extradural mass at the T9-10 levels with anterior displacement of the dural sac and cord. The patient was taken to surgery for evacuation of this spontaneous spinal epidural hematoma and was then found to have a bleeding time of 11.5 minutes (normal: 3 minutes). By the third postoperative day after garlic abstinence, the bleeding time returned to normal. This qualitative platelet disorder was surmised to result from his garlic ingestion.

Although the mechanism of action on hemostasis is different, concomitant use of garlic and warfarin is likely to result in excessive anticoagulation. This has been documented in two cases in which concomitant use of garlic and warfarin resulted in a doubling of "clotting times."[11]

Management Suggestions

Concomitant use of garlic and warfarin should be avoided. If the patient prevails in concomitant use, the clinician should closely monitor PT, INR, and bleeding time.

WARFARIN—GINGER

RELATED DRUGS

Abciximab	Enoxaparin
Alteplase	Eptifibatide
Anagrelide	Heparin
Anisindione	Lepirudin
Ardeparin	NSAIDs
Aspirin	Pentoxifylline
Cilostazol	Reteplase
Clopidogrel	Streptokinase
Dalteparin	Ticlodipine
Danaparoid	Tirofiban
Dicumarol	Urokinase
Dipyridamole	

Interaction Summary

Ginger might augment the anticoagulant activity of warfarin.

Discussion

Ginger has been found to inhibit platelet aggregation and alter arachidonic metabolism.[1] This translates into inhibition of thromboxane synthetase with decreased production of pro-

---

Rating Scale:

(1) Significant interaction

(2) Possibly significant interaction

(3) Interaction of relatively little significance

(4) Reported interaction that does not, in fact, exist or is insignificant

aggregatory thromboxane (TXA_2). Furthermore, it causes a rise in prostacyclin levels (PTI2), which inhibits aggregation.[1]

In a comparative study on platelet aggregation, onion and garlic extracts produced only mild inhibition (13% to 18%) of thromboxane B_2 formation, versus ginger extract, which reduced thromboxane B_2 formation by 73%.[2]

However, studies have not found any platelet effect when ginger is administered orally.[3-5] Nonetheless, if combined with other drugs that may affect platelet function, such as dipyridamole, ticlopidine, and clopidogrel, additive effects might occur. Additionally, if combined with other drugs that affect hemostasis, such as warfarin, dicumarol, and anisindione, increased anticoagulation might develop.

Management Suggestions

Theoretically, ginger may augment the anticoagulant and antiplatelet activities of other drugs. This, however, has not been observed (or monitored for) in humans. Patients taking both agents should have frequent monitoring of bleeding times initially.

WARFARIN—GINKGO

RELATED DRUGS

Abciximab	Enoxaparin
Alteplase	Eptifibatide
Anagrelide	Heparin
Anisindione	Lepirudin
Ardeparin	NSAIDs
Aspirin	Pentoxifylline
Cilostazol	Reteplase
Clopidogrel	Streptokinase
Dalteparin	Ticlodipine
Danaparoid	Tirofiban
Dicumarol	Urokinase
Dipyridamole	

Interaction Summary

Ginkgo may exacerbate the anticoagulant activity of warfarin and other agents that affect hemostasis.

Discussion

Several cases have been reported that suggest that ginkgo can adversely affect hemostasis. After 1 week of 40 mg ginkgo twice

Rating Scale:
(1) Significant interaction
(2) Possibly significant interaction
(3) Interaction of relatively little significance
(4) Reported interaction that does not, in fact, exist or is insignificant

daily, a 70-year-old man experienced spontaneous bleeding from the iris into the anterior chamber of the eye (hyphema).[1] The patient had also been taking one 325-mg tablet of aspirin daily for 3 years, but without incident; hence the authors attributed the hyphema to the ginkgo intake because of its temporal relationship.

A 61-year-old man taking *Ginkgo biloba*, 40 mg three to four times daily, developed subarachnoid hemorrhage after 6 months of use.[2] The patient's bleeding time was 6 minutes (normal: 1 to 3 minutes). The patient recovered uneventfully after discontinuing ginkgo and returned to a normal bleeding time of 3 minutes.

Another report documents spontaneous bilateral subdural hematomas associated with ginkgo in a 33-year-old Korean woman.[3] This patient had a 2-year history of chronic ginkgo ingestion of 120 mg daily. Her bleeding times were prolonged at 15 and 9.5 minutes (normal stated for this laboratory: 3 to 9 minutes). Upon discontinuation of ginkgo, her bleeding times decreased to within the normal range (6.5 minutes). The patient had no other risk factors; hence the authors concluded that the patient's presentation of subdural hematomas may have occurred at least in part due to the aberrant coagulopathy induced by ginkgo. It should be noted that bilateral subdural hematomas may occur without any history of head trauma or without known risk factors.[4] Furthermore, some clinicians dispute whether such a modest increase in bleeding time could lead to subdural bleeding.[4]

The apparent effect of ginkgo on hemostasis has been attributed to the content of ginkgolide B, a potent inhibitor of platelet-activating factor (PAF).[5] In a study of six healthy subjects aged 25 to 35 years, ginkgolide BN 52063 at doses of 80 and 120 mg resulted in an increase in the IC_{50} (i.e., the concentration of PAF needed to cause 50% of the maximum aggregatory response) from 4.1 ± 1.4 (SEM) nmol/L to 87.8 ± 50.4 (SEM) ($P < 0.001$).[5] It does not take much extrapolation to realize that there should be concern about the combination of ginkgo and warfarin.

Management Suggestions

Preliminary data suggest a temporal relationship between *Ginkgo biloba* ingestion and abnormalities in platelet function resulting in subdural hematomas and hyphema. To further the abnormalities in hemostasis with the addition of an anticoagulant such as warfarin is fraught with risk. Considering the narrow therapeutic window of warfarin, concomitant use is not recommended.

WARFARIN—
GINSENG (PANAX GINSENG)

Rating 2

RELATED DRUGS
Anisindione   Dicumarol

Interaction Summary

Panax ginseng might decrease the effectiveness of warfarin.

Discussion

A single case report exists detailing a decrease in warfarin's effectiveness with concomitant use of ginseng.[1] A 47-year-old man with a St. Jude–type mechanical heart valve had been stabilized on warfarin with an INR at 3.1. Two weeks after initiating ginseng, his INR declined to 1.5. No thrombotic episodes were noted. Ginseng was discontinued and the INR subsequently returned to 3.3. During this time the patient denied any change in drug therapy or dietary intake.

Panaxynol and ginsenosides Ro, Rg$_1$, and Rg$_2$ have been found to have antiplatelet effects, and may explain the occurrence outlined above.[2] However, a study in rats found no pharmacokinetic or pharmacodynamic interaction between warfarin and ginseng.[3]

Rating Scale:
(1) Significant interaction
(2) Possibly significant interaction
(3) Interaction of relatively little significance
(4) Reported interaction that does not, in fact, exist or is insignificant

Management Suggestions

Because warfarin has a narrow therapeutic window, it would be prudent for the patient not to use any other drugs, over-the-counter products, or herbal medicinals without first consulting a pharmacist or physician who is well versed in the use of herbal medicinals.

If a patient experiences a sudden decrease in the INR/PT despite continued therapy, the clinician should question the patient regarding ginseng use.

WARFARIN—PAPAYA EXTRACT

RELATED DRUGS

Anisindione   Heparin
Dicumarol

OTHER POTENTIALLY IMPLICATED SUPPLEMENTS

Boldo   Fenugreek

Interaction Summary

Concomitant use may result in elevated international normalized ratio (INR) and prothrombin time (PT).

Discussion

In a 5-year (1991-1995) toxicologic study in the United Kingdom, one case of warfarin interaction with papaya extract (containing papain) was encountered. A patient had been stabilized on warfarin but then started papaya extract for weight loss.[1] When admitted for cardiac surgery, his INR was 7.4. Both entities were discontinued with a subsequent fall of the INR to 2; surgery was then performed.

Rating Scale:
(1) Significant interaction
(2) Possibly significant interaction
(3) Interaction of relatively little significance
(4) Reported interaction that does not, in fact, exist or is insignificant

In addition, one case report suggests that a combination of the herbs boldo and fenugreek potentiated the effects of warfarin.[2]

Management Suggestions

Concomitant use of papain, boldo, or fenugreek with anticoagulants should be avoided.

WARFARIN—POLICOSANOL

RELATED DRUGS

Alteplase   Enoxaparin
Anisindione   Heparin
Ardeparin   Lepirudin
Dalteparin   Reteplase
Danaparoid   Streptokinase
Dicumarol   Urokinase

OTHER POTENTIALLY IMPLICATED SUPPLEMENTS

White willow   Saw palmetto

Interaction Summary

Policosanol has antiplatelet actions that might potentiate the anticoagulant effect of warfarin. White willow, a natural source of salicylates, might cause similar effects. Saw palmetto has been implicated in a case of intraoperative hemorrhage associated with increased bleeding times.

Discussion

Human trials have found that the supplement policosanol, used for hyperlipidemia, exhibits dose-dependent antiplatelet

---

Rating Scale:
(1)   Significant interaction
(2)   Possibly significant
      interaction

(3)   Interaction of relatively little
      significance
(4)   Reported interaction that
      does not, in fact, exist or is
      insignificant

actions.[1,2] This effect is comparable to that of aspirin, and combined treatment produces an additive effect.[3]

A 30-day, double-blind, placebo-controlled trial of 27 individuals with hypercholesterolemia found that policosanol at 10 mg/day markedly reduced platelet aggregation induced by collagen, low-dose ADP, or arachidonic acid.[1]

A double-blind, placebo-controlled study of 37 healthy volunteers found evidence of a dose-dependent effect.[2] In this trial, participants received placebo or policosanol, 10 mg/day for 7 days, following a 7-day placebo washout period. For a subsequent 7 days, the number of tablets was doubled, and then doubled again for a final 7 days. The results showed that antiplatelet effects in the treated group increased throughout the study, suggesting a dose-dependent relationship. However, a time effect cannot be ruled out.

A double-blind, placebo-controlled study of 43 healthy volunteers compared the effects of policosanol (20 mg/day), aspirin (100 mg/day), and combination therapy versus placebo.[3] The results showed that policosanol reduced ADP-induced platelet aggregation by 37%, epinephrine-induced aggregation by 21.9%, and collagen-induced aggregation by 40.5%. Aspirin reduced collagen-induced aggregation by 61.4% and epinephrine-induced aggregation by 21.9% but did not reduce ADP-induced aggregation. Combined therapy exhibited additive effects.

In addition, in one case report, use of the herb saw palmetto was associated with significantly increased bleeding time and intraoperative hemorrhage.[4]

Management Suggestions

Clinicians are advised to include policosanol and saw palmetto in their list of herbs and supplements to inquire about if a patient previously stabilized on warfarin begins to experience symptoms associated with increased anticoagulation. It would be prudent to obtain a bleeding time to ascertain if platelet function has been adversely affected, especially if the INR/PT is within the normal range.

WARFARIN—VINPOCETINE

Rating 3

RELATED DRUGS

Abciximab
Alteplase
Anagrelide
Anisindione
Ardeparin
Aspirin
Cilostazol
Clopidogrel
Dalteparin
Danaparoid
Dicumarol
Dipyridamole

Enoxaparin
Eptifibatide
Heparin
Lepirudin
NSAIDs
Pentoxifylline
Reteplase
Streptokinase
Ticlodipine
Tirofiban
Urokinase

Interaction Summary

Preliminary evidence suggests that vinpocetine might slightly impair the therapeutic effects of warfarin.

Discussion

Vinpocetine is a dietary supplement promoted for the treatment of age-related memory loss and impaired mental function. In a

---

Rating Scale:

(1) Significant interaction
(2) Possibly significant interaction

(3) Interaction of relatively little significance
(4) Reported interaction that does not, in fact, exist or is insignificant

24-day uncontrolled study, 18 male subjects received warfarin, 25 mg, on day 1. Prothrombin time (PT), warfarin plasma levels, and factor VII coagulation time were monitored on days 1 through 5.[1] Vinpocetine, 10 mg, was administered from day 6 to day 24. Another single dose of warfarin, 25 mg, was administered on day 20. AUC values of PT, drug plasma levels, and factor VII clotting time curves and appropriate C_{max} and t_{max} plasma levels of days 20 through 24 were compared with those of days 1 through 5. The results showed a tendency toward reduced anticoagulation.

Management Suggestions

As a precaution, consider monitoring coagulation parameters more frequently in patients taking vinpocetine with warfarin, and adjust the warfarin dose if needed.

WARFARIN—VITAMIN A

Rating 3

RELATED DRUGS

Anisindione   Dicumarol

OTHER POTENTIALLY IMPLICATED SUPPLEMENTS

Vitamin D

Interaction Summary

Vitamin A reportedly might increase the anticoagulant effects of warfarin, but there is little corroborating evidence.

Discussion

It has been reported that supplemental forms of vitamins A and D might increase the anticoagulant effects of warfarin.[1]

These reports are supported in the case of vitamin A by animal studies suggesting that vitamin A can increase the anticoagulant action of warfarin. There is little corroborating evidence for vitamin D.

Management Suggestions

Consider monitoring coagulation parameters more frequently in patients taking vitamin A with warfarin, and adjust the warfarin dose if needed. No such precautions appear necessary for vitamin D.

Rating Scale:
(1) Significant interaction
(2) Possibly significant interaction

(3) Interaction of relatively little significance
(4) Reported interaction that does not, in fact, exist or is insignificant

WARFARIN—VITAMIN C

Rating 3

RELATED DRUGS

Anisindione   Dicumarol

Interaction Summary

High-dose vitamin C (ascorbic acid) supplements might reduce warfarin's anticoagulant effects.

Discussion

Case reports suggest that vitamin C can reduce the anticoagulant effects of warfarin.[1-3] In one report, the patient was taking 1000 mg of vitamin C daily; another involved huge megadoses (about 16,000 mg daily). Animal studies, however, have not shown this effect for vitamin C.

Management Suggestions

Consider monitoring coagulation parameters more frequently in patients taking high-dose vitamin C with warfarin, and adjust the warfarin dose if needed.

Rating Scale:
(1) Significant interaction
(2) Possibly significant interaction

(3) Interaction of relatively little significance
(4) Reported interaction that does not, in fact, exist or is insignificant

WARFARIN—VITAMIN E

RELATED DRUGS

Alteplase	Enoxaparin
Anisindione	Heparin
Ardeparin	Lepirudin
Dalteparin	Reteplase
Danaparoid	Streptokinase
Dicumarol	Urokinase

Interaction Summary

Though a case report and an unpublished study suggest that vitamin E may potentiate warfarin's anticoagulant effect, a controlled study found no such interaction. However, the case report suggests that the time period of concurrent use might be a factor.

Discussion

A case report has given rise to concerns that vitamin E should not be combined with warfarin.[1] After 2 months of vitamin E supplementation at up to 1200 IU/day, a patient previously stabilized on warfarin presented with a markedly prolonged prothrombin time (PT) (36.6 seconds compared to control of 11.7 seconds) and bleeding. After restabilization, the patient was

---

Rating Scale:

(1) Significant interaction

(2) Possibly significant interaction

(3) Interaction of relatively little significance

(4) Reported interaction that does not, in fact, exist or is insignificant

rechallenged with vitamin E (800 IU/day) for a 7-week test period, during which platelet function tests remained within normal ranges. PT was affected by the fourth week and progressively increased over the next 2 weeks. Levels of vitamin K–dependent procoagulant factors declined, reaching their lowest point by the end of the sixth week. On day 42, multiple ecchymoses and a hematoma appeared. At that time, vitamin E was stopped, and 7 days later, coagulation parameters returned to baseline status and all clinical evidence of bleeding disappeared. A confounding factor is that the patient also was taking clofibrate, a drug known to enhance the bleeding effects of warfarin; however, the patient's bleeding status while taking warfarin and clofibrate, as well as other chronic medications, had been stabilized for 2 months before the vitamin E rechallenge.

In an unpublished study, three volunteers took a small daily dose of vitamin E (42 IU) for 30 days.[2] A 150-mg dose of dicumarol administered at the end of the vitamin E treatment period showed a marked increase in anticoagulant effect compared to the same dose given before vitamin E was started.

A synergistic interaction between vitamin E and warfarin seems logical, because vitamin E appears to inhibit platelet aggregation[3] and increase the risk of hemorrhagic stroke.[4] However, no interaction was seen in a 1996 double-blind study of 25 patients taking chronic warfarin therapy and given vitamin E at doses up to 1200 IU/day.[5] None of the 13 patients who took vitamin E at 800 or 1200 IU/day for 1 month had an increase in international normalized ratio (INR) that required a warfarin dose change. Interestingly, the two patients who met criteria for a possible or probable drug effect were taking placebo rather than vitamin E.

This study, though small and of short duration, suggests that doses of vitamin E up to 1200 IU/day can be used safely in patients receiving warfarin. However, it should be noted that, in the case report detailed above, a significant effect of vitamin E on PT did not occur until the fourth week, and the present study lasted only 4 weeks. As a precaution, it may be advisable to recheck the INR at selected intervals during the first 6 weeks after starting vitamin E.

Management Suggestions

Despite little evidence of an interaction, because of its potential consequences, it may be advisable to retest coagulation parameters at selected intervals during the first 6 weeks after initiating vitamin E supplementation in patients stabilized on warfarin.

WARFARIN—VITAMIN K

RELATED DRUGS

Anisindione   Dicumarol

Interaction Summary

Supplemental vitamin K, or changes in consumption of foods high in vitamin K, can alter the effect of therapy with oral anticoagulants such as warfarin.

Discussion

Dietary modifications involving foods high in vitamin K can alter the response to previously stabilized anticoagulant therapy.[1,2] For example, higher consumption of vitamin K–rich vegetables can impair the anticoagulant effect, and lower consumption can potentiate it. To avoid potential life-threatening complications, significant changes in diet, particularly involving foods rich in vitamin K, should be followed by redetermination of the international normalized ratio (INR).

Management Suggestions

The combination of vitamin K supplements and warfarin should be avoided except when oral or parenteral phytonadione (vita-

---

Rating Scale:
(1) Significant interaction
(2) Possibly significant interaction

(3) Interaction of relatively little significance
(4) Reported interaction that does not, in fact, exist or is insignificant

min K_1) is administered to overcome oral anticoagulant–induced hypoprothrombinemia. Patients on long-term warfarin therapy should be advised not to modify their diets without medical supervision. When dietary changes are made involving vitamin K–rich foods, the INR should be frequently monitored and the warfarin dose adjusted until anticoagulant stability has been restored.

ZIDOVUDINE—L-CARNITINE

Interaction Summary

Preliminary evidence suggests that the amino acid L-carnitine may diminish the mitochondrial toxicity associated with zidovudine (AZT) and other nucleoside analogs, exert independent positive effects on HIV infection parameters, and complement traditional chemotherapeutic regimens in HIV-infected patients.

Discussion

AZT therapy causes a mitochondrial myopathy, characterized by depletion of mitochondrial DNA and other destructive changes, that has been associated with a reduction of muscle carnitine levels.[1] Based on the observation that L-carnitine plays a major role in long-chain fatty acid transport and facilitates the beta-oxidation of fatty acids, it has been proposed as a treatment for these AZT side effects.[2]

In a human tissue study, myotubes prepared from muscle biopsies were exposed to various concentrations of AZT for up to 3 weeks.[2] One third of the flasks were treated with AZT alone, another third with AZT plus L-carnitine, and the remaining third were untreated. AZT at concentrations of 250 μM and higher was found to cause depopulation of Leu-19–positive myotubes and destructive changes in mitochondria, including accumulation of lipid droplets; in contrast, the addition of L-carnitine was found to in-

---

Rating Scale:

(1) Significant interaction

(2) Possibly significant interaction

(3) Interaction of relatively little significance

(4) Reported interaction that does not, in fact, exist or is insignificant

crease the number of Leu-19–positive myotubes, preserve the morphology of mitochondria, and prevent lipid accumulation.

Other preliminary evidence suggests that L-carnitine also may enhance immune function in persons with HIV. Eleven asymptomatic HIV-1–infected subjects, who refused antiretroviral treatment despite experiencing a progressive decline in CD4 counts, were treated with daily infusions of L-carnitine (6 g) for 4 months.[3] Immunologic and virologic measures and safety were monitored at the start of treatment and on days 15, 30, 90, and 150. L-Carnitine supplementation resulted in an increase in absolute CD4 counts, which was statistically significant on days 90 and 150 ($P = 0.010$ and ($P = 0.019$, respectively). A positive but not significant trend also was observed in the change in absolute counts of CD8 lymphocytes. Additionally, there was a decrease in the frequency of apoptotic CD4 and CD8 lymphocytes; the reduction was gradual but strongly significant ($P = 0.001$) at the end of the study compared to baseline. A strong reduction ($P = 0.001$) in cell-associated levels of ceramide, an endogenous mediator of Fas-triggered apoptosis that is related to the progression of HIV infection,[4] was also found at the end of the study. Another positive impact of L-carnitine was correction of disrupted mitochondrial transmembrane potential. This is an early irreversible step in the effector phase of apoptosis that allows identification of an additional pool of lymphocytes irreversibly committed to undergo apoptosis despite still lacking the morphologic features typical of apoptosis.[5] There was no clinically relevant change in HIV-1 viremia. L-Carnitine toxicity was not observed, and no dose reductions were necessary. These findings suggest that L-carnitine targets the immune system rather than the virus and further suggest that L-carnitine supplementation may complement antiretroviral therapy in the management of HIV-infected patients.

Management Suggestions

Based on these findings, L-carnitine supplementation may be worth trying in HIV-infected patients, whether or not they are taking AZT or other nucleoside analogs concurrently.

ZINC—AMILORIDE

Rating 3

RELATED DRUGS
Spironolactone   Triamterene

Interaction Summary

The potassium-sparing diuretic amiloride might significantly reduce zinc excretion, which could lead to zinc accumulation and possible toxicity. In contrast, triamterene, another potassium-sparing diuretic, appears to increase urinary zinc excretion.

Discussion

A literature review by Reyes et al. indicates that the potassium-sparing diuretic amiloride significantly reduces urinary zinc excretion at a dose of 10 mg, but not at a dose of 5 mg.[1] This raises the possibility that, at higher amiloride doses, zinc accumulation and possible toxicity could occur, particularly in the presence of alcoholism, renal insufficiency, or pregnancy. Interestingly, concurrent administration of amiloride, 5 mg, and the thiazide diuretic hydrochlorothiazide, 50 mg (which increases zinc urinary excretion), appears to maintain urinary zinc excretion within control ranges.

Rating Scale:
(1) Significant interaction
(2) Possibly significant interaction

(3) Interaction of relatively little significance
(4) Reported interaction that does not, in fact, exist or is insignificant

In contrast, a 2-week study reported that treatment with the potassium-sparing diuretic triamterene increased urinary zinc excretion by 18% compared to baseline.[2] However, zinc concentration in the urine did not change due to the diuretic-induced increase in urine volume. Whether this effect might be significant enough to promote zinc deficiency has not been assessed.

Management Suggestions

During treatment with amiloride, consider monitoring serum zinc levels and watch for signs of zinc toxicity such as flulike and central nervous system symptoms. High zinc levels also could lead to copper deficiency, with symptoms that include anemia and impaired immunity.[3]

Because marginal zinc deficiency is relatively common,[4-8] zinc supplementation at standard nutritional levels may be advisable during long-term triamterene use. Early symptoms of zinc deficiency include hypogeusia, hyposmia, sexual impotence, and delayed healing.

ZINC—CALCIUM CARBONATE

Interaction Summary

Calcium-containing antacids or calcium supplements might substantially decrease zinc absorption when taken with zinc supplements. However, eating a meal appears to mitigate this effect.

Discussion

Some studies have found significant effects of calcium supplements on zinc absorption, but others have found no effect. In one study, nine university students fasted and then took 4.5 mg of elemental zinc (as 20 mg zinc sulfate) with 600 mg of elemental calcium (as either 1500 mg calcium carbonate or 2850 mg calcium citrate).[1] The zinc tolerance test (ZTT) was used to quantitate zinc absorption. The plasma zinc AUC (mean ± SEM expressed as $Zn \times min/100$ g albumin) following coingestion of zinc with calcium carbonate (438.4 ± 129.0) and calcium citrate (308.0 ± 110.5) was significantly lower ($P < 0.017$) than that following ingestion of zinc alone (1561.7 ± 240), reflecting a 72% and 80% decline in zinc absorption associated with calcium carbonate and calcium citrate, respectively. The significance of this effect on zinc balance and retention, which is influenced by various homeostatic factors, is not clear, but it could assume clinical importance over the long term.

Rating Scale:

(1) Significant interaction

(2) Possibly significant interaction

(3) Interaction of relatively little significance

(4) Reported interaction that does not, in fact, exist or is insignificant

This study is unique in that it used physiologic doses of zinc and calcium comparable to the amounts found in meals; other studies have used much higher zinc doses.[2,3]

In contrast, in the presence of meals, zinc balance and retention appear to be unaffected by increases of either dietary sources of calcium or supplemental calcium.[4,5] A single-blind, placebo-controlled crossover study in 11 healthy postmenopausal women found no impairment of zinc absorption by calcium supplements taken with a standard test meal supplemented with 3.3 μCi of zinc-65.[4] Mean (SEM) zinc retention was 18.1% ± 1.0% with placebo and did not vary significantly with calcium carbonate or hydroxyapatite.

One possible explanation is that the ingestion of food is associated with a variety of complex interactions involving nutrients and digestive products that may affect nutrient absorption and disposition.

The mechanism by which supplemental calcium and zinc may interact is unknown, but experimental studies suggest that calcium might interfere with the uptake of zinc by the intestinal mucosa.[6]

Management Suggestions

To minimize any potential problems with this combination, administer calcium-containing antacids or calcium supplements 2 to 3 hours apart from zinc supplements.

ZINC—CAPTOPRIL

Rating 3

RELATED DRUGS

Benazepril	Lisinopril
Enalapril	Quinapril
Fosinopril	Ramipril

Interaction Summary

Zinc binds directly to structural groups on the ACE inhibitors captopril and enalapril, leading to a gradual depletion of tissue zinc and possible zinc deficiency.

Discussion

Captopril and enalapril possess a prominent zinc-binding moiety that binds to zinc in the active site of the ACE inhibitor.[1] The binding site for captopril contains a sulfhydryl group and that for enalapril contains a carboxyalkyl dipeptide group.

In a prospective study of the effects of ACE inhibitors on zinc levels, participants were divided into three groups according to agent: captopril ($n=16$), enalapril ($n=18$), or placebo ($n=10$).[1] Levels of zinc in serum, urine, and monocytes were similar for all three groups at baseline. When levels were measured again after 6 months, serum zinc showed no change from baseline in all three groups, and urinary zinc (μg/24-hour collection

---

Rating Scale:
(1) Significant interaction
(2) Possibly significant interaction

(3) Interaction of relatively little significance
(4) Reported interaction that does not, in fact, exist or is insignificant

period) had not changed in the placebo group. In contrast, 24-hour urinary zinc excretion was substantially higher in the captopril group (1244 ± 154 versus 461 ± 32, $P < 0.01$), and the enalapril group showed a small but statistically insignificant increase in urinary zinc loss. However, zinc concentrations in monocytes (nmol/mg protein)—an indicator of tissue zinc content—were significantly lower than at baseline in both the captopril (3.9 ± 1.2 versus 5.8 ± 2.4, $P < 0.01$) and enalapril (4.1 ± 2.3 versus 5.3 ± 2.5, $P < 0.04$) groups, and not in the placebo group. This last result indicates an ongoing loss of zinc from body tissues in the ACE inhibitor–treated groups during the 6-month study period.

A prior retrospective study assessing patients taking captopril ($n=6$), enalapril ($n=7$), or placebo ($n=9$) found that captopril therapy depleted zinc concentrations in red blood cells, also an indicator of tissue zinc stores, but enalapril did not.[2] However, this was a 3-month study, and it might be that enalapril takes longer to deplete tissue zinc.

These findings suggest that long-term treatment with captopril or enalapril—and possibly other ACE inhibitors—may result in a zinc deficiency. Additionally, the findings further confirm that diagnosing a zinc deficiency is not as straightforward as measuring zinc concentrations in the blood. It is possible, but not proven, that zinc deficiency might account for some of the side effects of ACE inhibitors such as taste disturbances, poor appetite, and paresthesias.

Management Suggestions

It may be reasonable to recommend zinc supplementation at nutritional doses to patients taking ACE inhibitors.

ZINC—
HYDROCHLOROTHIAZIDE

Rating 3

RELATED DRUGS

Bendroflumethiazide
Benzthiazide
Chlorothiazide
Chlorthalidone
Hydroflumethiazide
Indapamide

Methyclothiazide
Metolazone
Polythiazide
Quinethazone
Trichlormethiazide

Interaction Summary

Long-term use of thiazide diuretics may cause zinc depletion by increasing its urinary excretion. Clinically significant effects of this interaction are most likely in individuals with preexisting impaired zinc status.

Discussion

A literature review by Reyes et al. noted that thiazide diuretics, which act primarily in the first portion of the distal convoluted tubule in the nephron, have been found to increase urinary zinc excretion.[1] Both single-dose and long-term use of thiazides promote zinc loss.

Rating Scale:
(1) Significant interaction
(2) Possibly significant interaction

(3) Interaction of relatively little significance
(4) Reported interaction that does not, in fact, exist or is insignificant

The mechanism for the zinc-wasting effect of thiazide diuretics is poorly understood and may involve direct and hormone-mediated processes. Long-term use of thiazides can cause significant zinc depletion, especially in conditions that increase the risk of zinc depletion such as alcoholism, hepatic cirrhosis, renal disease, diabetes, gastrointestinal disorders, and pregnancy.[1,2]

Management Suggestions

During long-term thiazide diuretic treatment, supplementation with nutritional doses of zinc may be advisable. In addition, consider monitoring serum zinc levels and watch for early symptoms of zinc deficiency, which include hypogeusia and hyposmia, sexual impotence, delayed wound healing, skin disorders, and abnormal dark adaptation. Using minimal thiazide doses may be a simple way to help prevent diuretic-induced zinc depletion. A therapeutic option might be the use of low-dose amiloride (5 mg) concurrently with the thiazide, a combination that appears to help maintain zinc balance (see the **Zinc—Amiloride** article).

ZINC—ORAL CONTRACEPTIVES

Interaction Summary

Oral contraceptives (OCs) may reduce plasma zinc levels.

Discussion

Although there is disagreement, most studies have found that OCs (at least the high-estrogen type used at the time the studies were performed) may reduce plasma zinc levels.[1] The mechanism is unclear, as is the clinical significance of this finding.

Management Suggestions

Because marginal zinc deficiency is relatively common,[2-6] zinc supplementation at standard nutritional levels might be advisable for individuals taking OCs.

Rating Scale:

(1) Significant interaction

(2) Possibly significant interaction

(3) Interaction of relatively little significance

(4) Reported interaction that does not, in fact, exist or is insignificant

ZINC—ZIDOVUDINE

OTHER POTENTIALLY IMPLICATED SUPPLEMENTS

Copper   Vitamin B_{12}

Interaction Summary

Zidovudine (AZT) therapy may deplete zinc and copper; whether AZT might deplete vitamin B_{12} needs further clarification.

Discussion

A 1991 longitudinal study found significantly decreased mean plasma levels of zinc and copper in AZT-treated participants after 12 months of drug therapy.[1] Of 37 HIV-1–seropositive participants, 15 were treated with AZT (500 to 1200 mg/day) and 22 served as untreated, CD4-matched controls. Plasma nutrient levels were similar in both groups prior to AZT administration. After 12 months of AZT treatment, a large proportion (67%) of AZT-treated patients exhibited zinc deficiency compared to 24% of the untreated group, with the difference between the two groups being statistically significant ($P < 0.03$). AZT-treated patients showed a significant ($P < 0.03$) decline in zinc levels (mean $\pm$ SD: 0.75 ± 0.23 µg/ml) compared to baseline (0.86 ± 0.1 µg/ml). Plasma zinc remained stable in the untreated group (0.81 ± 0.1 µg/ml; baseline: 0.86 ± 0.3; $P < 0.03$). Additionally, mean plasma copper levels decreased

---

Rating Scale:

(1) Significant interaction

(2) Possibly significant interaction

(3) Interaction of relatively little significance

(4) Reported interaction that does not, in fact, exist or is insignificant

significantly ($P < 0.05$) in AZT-treated patients from 0.96 ± 0.14 to 0.86 ± 0.14 μg/ml, whereas copper levels in the untreated group did not change. Zinc depletion in the drug-treated patients occurred despite adequate zinc intake. Adequate zinc levels were associated with enhanced lymphocyte responsiveness in the treated patients, suggesting that zinc was particularly important in maintaining immune function in this group. Furthermore, because AZT requires the zinc-dependent enzyme thymidine kinase for conversion to its active triphosphate form,[2] zinc deficiency may diminish drug effectiveness.

The importance of zinc in immune function is well known. A 1995 study found that zinc sulfate supplementation decreased the number of opportunistic infections in HIV-infected persons treated with AZT.[3] The zinc supplement was administered orally at a daily dose of 200 mg for 30 days to AZT-treated stage III patients with generalized lymphadenopathy ($n=17$) and stage IV subgroup C1 patients ($n=12$). Controls consisted of stage III patients with generalized lymphadenopathy ($n=18$) and stage IV subgroup C1 patients ($n=10$), who were treated with AZT alone. Zinc supplementation was associated with positive effects on body weight, number of CD4+ cells, and plasma levels of active zinc-bound thymulin hormone. Furthermore, the frequency of opportunistic infectious episodes during the 24-month follow-up was reduced in zinc-supplemented stage IV C1 subjects compared to control (11 versus 25) and was delayed in zinc-supplemented stage III patients (1/24 months versus 13/24 months). The zinc benefit was observed for infections due to *Pneumocystis carinii* and *Candida* but not for cytomegalovirus and *Toxoplasma* infections.

Decreased vitamin B_{12} (cobalamin) levels frequently are found in HIV disease, particularly among those treated with AZT. Paltiel et al. conducted a cross-sectional survey of 200 HIV-infected patients, including a prospective follow-up in a subgroup of subjects before and after initiation of AZT therapy.[4] Subnormal serum B_{12} levels were found in 61 subjects (30.5%), and B_{12}-deficient patients were more likely to be taking AZT ($P = 0.007$).

Malabsorption of B_{12} as evidenced by abnormal Schilling tests was found to be more likely among patients with more advanced HIV disease or gastrointestinal symptoms but was not necessarily associated with low B_{12} levels. Despite a high prevalence of subnormal B_{12} levels in this population, none of the data support a hypothesis that selective tissue B_{12} deficiency occurs. Further investigation is needed to clarify a possible relationship between AZT therapy and the increased incidence of low serum B_{12} levels found in HIV-infected patients.

Management Suggestions

Based on these findings, monitoring of nutritional status during AZT chemotherapeutic regimens would be advisable, as well as supplementation with zinc, copper, and vitamin B_{12} when indicated. Because HIV infection itself may adversely affect the absorption of many nutrients, adequate nutrition in general is important.

ZOLPIDEM—5-HTP

Rating 2

OTHER POTENTIALLY IMPLICATED SUPPLEMENTS

L-Tryptophan   St. John's wort

Interaction Summary

Several case reports suggest that the risk of zolpidem-induced visual hallucinations may be increased when the drug is combined with agents that enhance serotonin activity.

Discussion

Over a 2-year period, the Washington Poison Center received five reports of prolonged visual hallucinations associated with the hypnotic agent zolpidem.[1] All five patients reported visual hallucinations lasting from 1 to 7 hours soon after taking zolpidem. Most had been taking the drug for less than a week, and all five were concurrently taking an antidepressant (sertraline, desipramine, fluoxetine, bupropion, or venlafaxine). Combining these cases with five previously published reports revealed that nine of the ten patients with persistent symptoms were concurrently taking antidepressants that inhibit serotonin reuptake. Though zolpidem has no known effect on serotonin, these findings suggest that the reported adverse reaction might be the

Rating Scale:

(1) Significant interaction

(2) Possibly significant interaction

(3) Interaction of relatively little significance

(4) Reported interaction that does not, in fact, exist or is insignificant

result of a pharmacodynamic interaction between serotonin re-uptake inhibition and zolpidem.

Management Suggestions

5-HTP and L-tryptophan are both serotonin precursors, and St. John's wort is thought to raise serotonin levels. Based on the case reports, patients taking zolpidem should be advised to avoid these supplements.

REFERENCES

5-HTP—Levodopa/Carbidopa

1. Joly P, Lampert A, Thomine E, et al. Development of pseudobullous morphea and scleroderma-like illness during therapy with L-5-hydroxytryptophan and carbidopa. *J Am Acad Dermatol.* 1991; 25:332-333.

2. Sternberg EM, Van Woert MH, Young SN, et al. Development of a scleroderma-like illness during therapy with L-5-hydroxytryptophan and carbidopa. *N Engl J Med.* 1980;303:782-787.

ACE Inhibitors—Iron

1. Campbell NR, Hasinoff BB. Iron supplements: a common cause of drug interactions. *Br J Clin Pharmacol.* 1991;31:251-255.

ACE Inhibitors—Potassium

1. Good CB, McDermott L, McCloskey B. Diet and serum potassium in patients on ACE inhibitors [letter]. *JAMA.* 1995;274:538.

2. Burnakis TG, Mioduch HJ. Combined therapy with captopril and potassium supplementation: a potential for hyperkalemia. *Arch Intern Med.* 1984;144:2371-2372.

3. Grossman A, Eckland D, Price P, et al. Captopril: reversible renal failure with severe hyperkalaemia [letter]. *Lancet.* 1980;1:712.

4. Warren SE, O'Conner DT. Hyperkalemia resulting from captopril administration. *JAMA.* 1980;244:2551-2552.

5. Stoltz ML, Andrews CE Jr. Severe hyperkalemia during very-low-calorie diets and angiotensin converting enzyme use [letter]. *JAMA.* 1990;264:2737-2738.

Acetaminophen—Vitamin C

1. Houston JB, Levy G. Drug biotransformation interactions in man VI: acetaminophen and ascorbic acid. *J Pharm Sci.* 1976; 65:1218-1221.

Alprazolam—Kava

1. Almeida JC, Grimsley EW. Coma from the health food store: interaction between kava and alprazolam [letter]. *Ann Intern Med.* 1996;125:940-941.

2. Jussofie A, Schmiz A, Hiemke C. Kavapyrone enriched extract from *Piper methysticum* as modulator of the GABA binding site in different regions of rat brain. *Psychopharmacology (Berl)*. 1994; 116:469-474.

3. Davies LP, Drew CA, Duffield P, et al. Kava pyrones and resin: studies on GABA$_A$, GABA$_B$ and benzodiazepine binding sites in rodent brain. *Pharmacol Toxicol*. 1992;71:120-126.

4. Boonen G, Haberlein H. Influence of genuine kavapyrone enantiomers on the GABA-A binding site. *Planta Med*. 1998;64: 504-506.

5. Boonen G, Ferger B, Kuschinsky K, et al. In vivo effects of the kavapyrones (+)–dihydromethysticin and (±)–kavain on dopamine, 3,4-dihydroxyphenylacetic acid, serotonin and 5-hydroxyindoleacetic acid levels in striatal and cortical brain regions. *Planta Med*. 1998;64:507-510.

Aluminum Hydroxide—Calcium Citrate

1. Nolan CR, Califano JR, Butzin CA. Influence of calcium acetate or calcium citrate on intestinal aluminum absorption. *Kidney Int*. 1990;38:937-941.

2. [No authors listed]. Preliminary findings suggest calcium citrate supplements may raise aluminum levels in blood, urine. *Fam Pract News*. 1992;22:74-75.

3. Walker JA, Sherman RA, Cody RP. The effect of oral bases on enteral aluminum absorption. *Arch Intern Med*. 1990;150: 2037-2039.

4. Weberg R, Berstad A. Gastrointestinal absorption of aluminium from single doses of aluminium containing antacids in man. *Eur J Clin Invest*. 1986;16:428-432.

5. Slanina P, Frech W, Bernhardson A, et al. Influence of dietary factors on aluminium absorption and retention in the brain and bone of rats. *Acta Pharmacol Toxicol (Copenh)*. 1985;56:331-336.

Amiodarone—Chaparral

1. Alderman S, Kailas S, Goldfarb S, et al. Cholestatic hepatitis after ingestion of chaparral leaf: confirmation by endoscopic retrograde cholangiopancreatography and liver biopsy. *J Clin Gastroenterol*. 1994;19:242-247.

2. [No authors listed]. From the Centers for Disease Control and Prevention. Chaparral-induced toxic hepatitis—California and Texas, 1992. *JAMA.* 1992;268:3295, 3298.

3. Gordon DW, Rosenthal G, Hart J, et al. Chaparral ingestion. The broadening spectrum of liver injury caused by herbal medications. *JAMA.* 1995;273:489-490.

4. Katz M, Saibil F. Herbal hepatitis: subacute hepatic necrosis secondary to chaparral leaf. *J Clin Gastroenterol.* 1990;12:203-206.

5. Smith BC, Desmond PV. Acute hepatitis induced by ingestion of the herbal medication chaparral [letter]. *Aust N Z J Med.* 1993; 23:526.

6. Sheikh NM, Philen RM, Love LA. Chaparral-associated hepatotoxicity. *Arch Intern Med.* 1997;157:913-919.

7. Agarwal R, Wang ZY, Bik DP, et al. Nordihydroguaiaretic acid, an inhibitor of lipoxygenase, also inhibits cytochrome P-450–mediated monooxygenase activity in rat epidermal and hepatic microsomes. *Drug Metab Dispos.* 1991;19:620-624.

8. Salari H, Braquet P, Borgeat P. Comparative effects of indomethacin, acetylenic acids, 15-hete, nordihydroguaiaretic acid and bw755c on the metabolism of arachidonic acid in human leukocytes and platelets. *Prostaglandins Leukot Med.* 1984;13: 53-60.

9. Jim LK, Gee JP. Adverse effects of drugs on the liver. In: Young LY, Koda-Kimble MA, eds. *Applied Therapeutics: The Clinical Use of Drugs.* Vancouver, Wash: Applied Therapeutics, Inc.; 1995;26.1-26.17.

Aspirin—Fish Oil

1. Harris WS. Dietary fish oil and blood lipids. *Curr Opin Lipidol.* 1996;7:3-7.

2. Leaf A, Jorgensen MB, Jacobs AK, et al. Do fish oils prevent restenosis after coronary angioplasty? *Circulation.* 1994;90:2248-2257.

Aspirin—Policosanol

1. Cheema P, El-Mefty O, Jazieh AR. Intraoperative haemorrhage associated with the use of extract of saw palmetto herb: a case report and review of literature. *J Intern Med.* 2001;250:167-169.

2. Arruzazabala ML, Mas R, Molina V, et al. Effect of policosanol on platelet aggregation in type II hypercholesterolemic patients. *Int J Tissue React.* 1998;20:119-124.

3. Arruzazabala ML, Valdes S, Mas R, et al. Effect of policosanol successive dose increases on platelet aggregation in healthy volunteers. *Pharmacol Res.* 1996;34:181-185.

4. Arruzazabala ML, Valdes S, Mas R, et al. Comparative study of policosanol, aspirin and the combination therapy policosanol-aspirin on platelet aggregation in healthy volunteers. *Pharmacol Res.* 1997;36:293-297.

Aspirin—Vitamin E

1. White JG, Rao GH, Gerrard JM. Effects of nitroblue tetrazolium and vitamin E on platelet ultrastructure, aggregation, and secretion. *Am J Pathol.* 1977;88:387-402.

2. Liede KE, Haukka JK, Saxen LM, et al. Increased tendency towards gingival bleeding caused by joint effect of alpha-tocopherol supplementation and acetylsalicylic acid. *Ann Med.* 1998;30:542-546.

3. Steiner M, Glantz M, Lekos A. Vitamin E plus aspirin compared with aspirin alone in patients with transient ischemic attacks. *Am J Clin Nutr.* 1995;62(6 suppl):1381S-1384S.

4. Leppala JM, Virtamo J, Fogelholm R, et al. Controlled trial of alpha-tocopherol and beta-carotene supplements on stroke incidence and mortality in male smokers. *Arterioscler Thromb Vasc Biol.* 2000;20:230-235.

Beta-Blockers—Calcium

1. Kirch W, Schafer-Korting M, Axthelm T, et al. Interaction of atenolol with furosemide and calcium and aluminum salts. *Clin Pharmacol Ther.* 1981;30:429-435.

Biotin—Carbamazepine

1. Krause KH, Bonjour JP, Berlit P, et al. Biotin status of epileptics. *Ann N Y Acad Sci.* 1985;447:297-313.

2. Said HM, Redha R, Nylander W. Biotin transport in the human intestine: inhibition by anticonvulsant drugs. *Am J Clin Nutr.* 1989;49:127-131.

Bromocriptine—Chasteberry

1. Jarry H, Leonhardt S, Gorkow C, et al. In vitro prolactin but not LH and FSH release is inhibited by compounds in extracts of *Agnus castus:* direct evidence for a dopaminergic principle by the dopamine receptor assay. *Exp Clin Endocrinol.* 1994;102:448-454.

2. Winterhoff H. Medicinal plants with endocrine efficacy. Effects on thyroid and ovary function [translated from German]. *Z Phytother.* 1993;14:83-94.

3. Milewicz A, Gejdel E, Sworen H, et al. *Vitex agnus castus* extract in the treatment of luteal phase defects due to latent hyperprolactinemia. Results of a randomized placebo-controlled double-blind study [translated from German]. *Arzneimittelforschung.* 1993;43:752-756.

Calcium—Corticosteroids

1. Buckley LM, Leib ES, Cartularo KS, et al. Calcium and vitamin D3 supplementation prevents bone loss in the spine secondary to low-dose corticosteroids in patients with rheumatoid arthritis: a randomized, double-blind, placebo-controlled study. *Ann Intern Med.* 1996;125:961-968.

2. Adachi JD, Bensen WG, Bianchi F, et al. Vitamin D and calcium in the prevention of corticosteroid induced osteoporosis: a 3 year followup. *J Rheumatol.* 1996;23:995-1000.

3. Homik J, Suarez-Almazor ME, Shea B, et al. Calcium and vitamin D for corticosteroid-induced osteoporosis. *Cochrane Database Syst Rev.* 2000;30:1-9.

4. Dykman TR, Haralson KM, Gluck OS, et al. Effect of oral 1,25-dihydroxyvitamin D and calcium on glucocorticoid-induced osteopenia in patients with rheumatic diseases. *Arthritis Rheum.* 1984;27:1336-1343.

Calcium—Digoxin

1. Kupfer S, Kosovsky JD. Effects of cardiac glycosides on renal tubular transport of calcium, magnesium, inorganic phosphate, and glucose in the dog. *J Clin Invest.* 1965;44:1132-1143.

Calcium—Phenytoin

1. Wahl TO, Gobuty AH, Lukert BP. Long-term anticonvulsant therapy and intestinal calcium absorption. *Clin Pharmacol Ther.* 1981;30:506-512.

2. Weinstein RS, Bryce GF, Sappington LJ, et al. Decreased serum ionized calcium and normal vitamin D metabolite levels with anticonvulsant drug treatment. *J Clin Endocrinol Metab.* 1984;58: 1003-1009.

3. Carter BL, Garnett WR, Pellock JM, et al. Effect of antacids on phenytoin bioavailability. *Ther Drug Monit.* 1981;3:333-340.

4. McElnay JC, Uprichard G, Collier PS. The effect of activated dimethicone and a proprietary antacid preparation containing this agent on the absorption of phenytoin. *Br J Clin Pharmacol.* 1982; 13:501-505.

Calcium—Thiazide Diuretics

1. Lemann J Jr, Gray RW, Maierhofer WJ, et al. Hydrochlorothiazide inhibits bone resorption in men despite experimentally elevated serum 1,25-dihydroxyvitamin D concentrations. *Kidney Int.* 1985;28:951-958.

2. Riis B, Christiansen C. Actions of thiazide on vitamin D metabolism: a controlled therapeutic trial in normal women early in the postmenopause. *Metabolism.* 1985;34:421-424.

3. Crowe M, Wollner L, Griffiths RA. Hypercalcaemia following vitamin D and thiazide therapy in the elderly. *Practitioner.* 1984;228: 312-313.

4. Gora ML, Seth SK, Bay WH, et al. Milk-alkali syndrome associated with use of chlorothiazide and calcium carbonate. *Clin Pharm.* 1989;8:227-229.

Carbamazepine—Grapefruit Juice

1. Bailey DG, Malcolm J, Arnold O, et al. Grapefruit juice–drug interactions. *Br J Clin Pharmacol.* 1998;46:101-110.

2. *A to Z Drug Facts* [book on CD-ROM]. 2nd ed. St. Louis, Mo: Facts and Comparisons; 2000.

3. Fuhr U. Drug interactions with grapefruit juice. Extent, probable mechanism and clinical relevance. *Drug Saf.* 1998;18:251-272.

4. Takanaga H, Ohnishi A, Murakami H, et al. Relationship between time after intake of grapefruit juice and the effect on pharmacokinetics and pharmacodynamics of nisoldipine in healthy subjects. *Clin Pharmacol Ther.* 2000;67:201-214.

5. Budzinski JW, Foster BC, Vandenhoek S, et al. An *in vitro* evaluation of human cytochrome P450 3A4 inhibition by selected commercial herbal extracts and tinctures. *Phytomedicine.* 2000;7: 273-282.

Carbamazepine—Nicotinamide (Niacinamide)

1. Bourgeois BF, Dodson WE, Ferrendelli JA. Interactions between primidone, carbamazepine, and nicotinamide. *Neurology.* 1982;32: 1122-1126.

Carnitine—Valproic Acid

1. De Vivo DC, Bohan TP, Coulter DL, et al. L-Carnitine supplementation in childhood epilepsy: current perspectives. *Epilepsia.* 1998;39:1216-1225.

2. Camina MF, Rozas I, Gomez M, et al. Short-term effects of administration of anticonvulsant drugs on free carnitine and acyl-carnitine in mouse serum and tissues. *Br J Pharmacol.* 1991;103: 1179-1183.

3. Matsuda I, Ohtani Y. Carnitine status in Reye and Reye-like syndromes. *Pediatr Neurol.* 1986;2:90-94.

4. Freeman JM, Vining EPG, Cost S, et al. Does carnitine administration improve the symptoms attributed to anticonvulsant medications? A double-blinded, crossover study. *Pediatrics.* 1994; 93:893-895.

5. Zelnik N, Fridkis I, Gruener N. Reduced carnitine and anti-epileptic drugs: cause relationship or co-existence? *Acta Paediatr.* 1995;84:93-95.

6. Rodriguez-Segade S, de la Pena CA, Tutor JC, et al. Carnitine deficiency associated with anticonvulsant therapy. *Clin Chim Acta.* 1989;181:175-181.

7. Hug G, McGraw CA, Bates SR, et al. Reduction of serum carnitine concentrations during anticonvulsant therapy with phenobarbital, valproic acid, phenytoin, and carbamazepine in children. *J Pediatr.* 1991;119:799-802.

8. Chung S, Choi J, Hyun T, et al. Alterations in the carnitine metabolism in epileptic children treated with valproic acid. *J Korean Med Sci.* 1997;12:553-558.

9. Coulter DL. Carnitine deficiency: a possible mechanism for valproate hepatotoxicity [letter]. *Lancet.* 1984;1:689.

10. Melegh B, Pap M, Morava E, et al. Carnitine-dependent changes of metabolic fuel consumption during long-term treatment with valproic acid. *J Pediatr.* 1994;125:317-321.

Chromium—Calcium Carbonate

1. Seaborn CD, Stoecker BJ. Effects of antacid or ascorbic acid on tissue accumulation and urinary excretion of 51-chromium. *Nutr Res.* 1990;10:1401-1407.

2. Mertz W. Chromium in human nutrition: a review. *J Nutr.* 1993; 123:626-633.

Ciprofloxacin—Fennel

1. Zhu M, Wong PY, Li RC. Effect of oral administration of fennel *(Foeniculum vulgare)* on ciprofloxacin absorption and disposition in the rat. *J Pharm Pharmacol.* 1999;51:1391-1396.

Clomipramine—SAMe

1. Iruela LM, Minguez L, Merino J, et al. Toxic interaction of S-adenosylmethionine and clomipramine [letter]. *Am J Psychiatry.* 1993;150:522.

2. Hernandez AF, Montero N, Pla A, et al. Fatal moclobemide overdose or death caused by serotonin syndrome? *J Food Prot.* 1995; 40:128-130.

3. Mason BJ, Blackburn KH. Possible serotonin syndrome associated with tramadol and sertraline coadministration. *Ann Pharmacother.* 1997;31:175-177.

Clonidine—Yohimbe (Source of Yohimbine)

1. *Review of Natural Products.* St. Louis, Mo: Facts and Comparisons; 1993: Yohimbe monograph.

2. Goldstein DS, Grossman E, Listwak S, et al. Sympathetic reactivity during a yohimbine challenge test in essential hypertension. *Hypertension.* 1991;18(5 suppl):III40-III48.

3. Murburg MM, Villacres EC, Ko GN, et al. Effects of yohimbine in human sympathetic nervous system function. *J Clin Endocrinol Metab.* 1991;73:861-865.

4. Grossman E, Rosenthal T, Peleg E, et al. Oral yohimbine increases blood pressure and sympathetic nervous outflow in hypertensive patients. *J Cardiovasc Pharmacol.* 1993;22:22-26.

5. Charney DS, Heninger GR, Breier A. Noradrenergic function in panic anxiety: effects of yohimbine in healthy subjects and patients with agoraphobia and panic disorder. *Arch Gen Psychiatry.* 1984;41:751-763.

6. Musso NR, Vergassola C, Pende A, et al. Yohimbine effects on blood pressure and plasma catecholamines in human hypertension. *Am J Hypertens.* 1995;8:565-571.

7. Hoffmann BB, Lefkowitz RJ. Catecholamines, sympathomimetic drugs, and adrenergic receptor antagonists. In: Hardman JG, Limbird LE, eds. *Goodman & Gilman's The Pharmacological Basis of Therapeutics.* 9th ed. New York, NY: McGraw-Hill, Health Professions Division; 1996:100-248.

8. Charney DS, Heninger GR, Sternberg DE. Assessment of alpha$_2$ adrenergic autoreceptor function in humans: effects of oral yohimbine. *Life Sci.* 1982;30:2033-2041.

9. De Smet PA, Smeets OS. Potential risks of health food products containing yohimbe extracts [letter]. *BMJ.* 1994;309:958.

10. Charney DS, Heninger GR, Sternberg DE. Yohimbine induced anxiety and increased noradrenergic function in humans: effects of diazepam and clonidine. *Life Sci.* 1983;33:19-29.

11. Charney DS, Breier A, Jatlow PI, et al. Behavioral, biochemical, and blood pressure responses to alprazolam in healthy subjects: interactions with yohimbine. *Psychopharmacology.* 1986;88:133-140.

12. Lecrubier Y, Puech AJ, Des Lauriers A. Favourable effects of yohimbine on clomipramine-induced orthostatic hypotension: a double-blind study. *Br J Clin Pharmacol.* 1981;12:90-93.

13. Charney DS, Price LH, Heninger GR. Desipramine-yohimbine combination treatment of refractory depression: implications for the beta-adrenergic receptor hypothesis of antidepressant action. *Arch Gen Psychiatry.* 1986;43:1155-1161.

14. Lacomblez L, Bensimon G, Isnard F, et al. Effect of yohimbine on blood pressure in patients with depression and orthostatic hypotension induced by clomipramine. *Clin Pharmacol Ther.* 1989;45:241-251.

Coenzyme Q$_{10}$—Acetohexamide

1. Kishi T, Kishi H, Watanabe T, et al. Bioenergetics in clinical medicine. XI. Studies on coenzyme Q and diabetes mellitus. *J Med.* 1976;7:307-321.

2. Singh RB, Niaz MA, Rastogi SS, et al. Effect of hydrosoluble coenzyme Q10 on blood pressures and insulin resistance in hypertensive patients with coronary artery disease. *J Hum Hypertens.* 1999;13:203-208.

Coenzyme Q$_{10}$—Chlorpromazine

1. Mortensen SA, Vadhanavikit S, Muratsu K, et al. Coenzyme Q10: clinical benefits with biochemical correlates suggesting a scientific breakthrough in the management of chronic heart failure. *Int J Tissue React.* 1990;12:155-162.

2. Folkers K. Basic chemical research on coenzyme Q10 and integrated clinical research on therapy of diseases. *Biomed Clin Aspects Coenzyme Q.* 1985;5:457-478.

3. Kishi T, Makino K, Okamoto T, et al. Inhibition of myocardial respiration by psychotherapeutic drugs and prevention by coenzyme Q. *Biomed Clin Aspects Coenzyme Q.* 1980;2:139-157.

Coenzyme Q$_{10}$—Lovastatin

1. Ghirlanda G, Oradei A, Manto A, et al. Evidence of plasma CoQ10-lowering effect by HMG-CoA reductase inhibitors: a double-blind, placebo-controlled study. *J Clin Pharmacol.* 1993;33:226-229.

2. Mortensen SA, Leth A, Agner E, et al. Dose-related decrease of serum coenzyme Q10 during treatment with HMG-CoA reductase inhibitors. *Mol Aspects Med.* 1997;18(suppl):S137-S144.

3. Mortensen SA, Vadhanavikit S, Muratsu K, et al. Coenzyme Q10: clinical benefits with biochemical correlates suggesting a scientific breakthrough in the management of chronic heart failure. *Int J Tissue React.* 1990;12:155-162.

4. Folkers K, Langsjoen P, Willis R, et al. Lovastatin decreases coenzyme Q levels in humans. *Proc Natl Acad Sci U S A.* 1990;87:8931-8934.

5. Bargossi AM, Battino M, Gaddi A, et al. Exogenous CoQ10 preserves plasma ubiquinone levels in patients treated with 3-hydroxy-3-methylglutaryl coenzyme A reductase inhibitors. *Int J Clin Lab Res.* 1994;24:171-176.

Coenzyme Q₁₀—Propranolol

1. Mortensen SA, Vadhanavikit S, Muratsu K, et al. Coenzyme Q10: clinical benefits with biochemical correlates suggesting a scientific breakthrough in the management of chronic heart failure. *Int J Tissue React.* 1990;12:155-162.

2. Kishi H, Kishi T, Folkers K. Bioenergetics in clinical medicine. III. Inhibition of coenzyme Q10-enzymes by clinically used antihypertensive drugs. *Res Commun Chem Pathol Pharmacol.* 1975;12:533-540.

3. Hamada M, Kazatain Y, Ochi T, et al. Correlation between serum CoQ10 level and myocardial contractility in hypertensive patients. *Biomed Clin Aspects Coenzyme Q.* 1984;4:263-270.

Copper—Oral Contraceptives

1. Milne DB, Johnson PE. Assessment of copper status: effect of age and gender on reference ranges in healthy adults. *Clin Chem.* 1993;39:883-887.

2. Newhouse IJ, Clement DB, Lai C. Effects of iron supplementation and discontinuation on serum copper, zinc, calcium, and magnesium levels in women. *Med Sci Sports Exerc.* 1993;25:562-571.

3. Berg G, Kohlmeier L, Brenner H. Effect of oral contraceptive progestins on serum copper concentration. *Eur J Clin Nutr.* 1998;52:711-715.

4. Reunanen A, Knekt P, Marniemi J, et al. Serum calcium, magnesium, copper and zinc and risk of cardiovascular death. *Eur J Clin Nutr.* 1996;50:431-437.

5. Salonen JT, Salonen R, Korpela H, et al. Serum copper and the risk of acute myocardial infarction: a prospective population study in men in eastern Finland. *Am J Epidemiol.* 1991;134:268-276.

Corticosteroids—Chromium

1. Ravina A, Slezak L, Mirsky N, et al. Control of steroid-induced diabetes with supplemental chromium. *J Trace Elem Exp Med.* 1999;12:375-378.

2. Anderson RA, Cheng N, Bryden NA, et al. Elevated intakes of supplemental chromium improve glucose and insulin variables in individuals with type 2 diabetes. *Diabetes.* 1997;46:1786-1791.

3. Ravina A, Slezack L. Chromium in the treatment of clinical diabetes mellitus [translated from Hebrew]. *Harefuah.* 1993;125:142-145.

4. Jovanovic L, Gutierrez M, Peterson CM. Chromium supplementation for women with gestational diabetes mellitus. *J Trace Elem Exp Med.* 1999;12:91-97.

5. Rabinowitz MB, Gonick HC, Levin SR, et al. Effects of chromium and yeast supplements on carbohydrate and lipid metabolism in diabetic men. *Diabetes Care.* 1983;6:319-327.

Cyclosporine—Echinacea

1. Dorn M, Knick E, Lewith G. Placebo-controlled double-blind study of *Echinacea pallidae* radix in upper respiratory tract infections. *Complement Ther Med.* 1997;5:40-42.

2. Hoheisel O, Sandberg M, Bertram S, et al. Echinagard treatment shortens the course of the common cold: a double-blind placebo-controlled clinical trial. *Eur J Clin Res.* 1997;9:261-268.

3. Wustenberg P, Henneicke-von Zepelin H-H, Kohler G, et al. Efficacy and mode of action of an immunomodulator herbal preparation containing echinacea, wild indigo, and white cedar. *Adv Ther.* 1999;16:51-70.

4. Stimpel M, Proksch A, Wagner H, et al. Macrophage activation and induction of macrophage cytotoxicity by purified polysaccharide fractions from the plant *Echinacea purpurea. Infect Immun.* 1984;46:845-849.

5. Melchart D, Linde K, Worku F, et al. Results of five randomized studies on the immunomodulatory activity of preparations of *Echinacea. J Altern Complement Med.* 1995;1:145-160.

Cyclosporine—Ipriflavone

1. Alexandersen P, Toussaint A, Christiansen C, et al. Ipriflavone in the treatment of postmenopausal osteoporosis: a randomized controlled trial. *JAMA.* 2001;285:1482-1488.

2. Agnusdei D, Bufalino L. Efficacy of ipriflavone in established osteoporosis and long-term safety. *Calcif Tissue Int.* 1997;61(suppl 1):S23-S27.

Cyclosporine—St. John's Wort

1. Guengerich FP. Cytochrome P-450 3A4: regulation and role in drug metabolism. *Annu Rev Pharmacol Toxicol.* 1999;39:1-17.

2. Ruschitzka F, Meier PJ, Turina M, et al. Acute heart transplant rejection due to St. John's wort [letter]. *Lancet.* 2000;355:548-549.

3. Johne A, Brockmuller J, Bauer S, et al. Pharmacokinetic interaction of digoxin with an herbal extract from St. John's wort *(Hypericum perforatum). Clin Pharmacol Ther.* 1999;66:338-345.

4. Breidenbach T, Hoffmann MW, Becker T, et al. Drug interaction of St John's wort with cyclosporin [letter]. *Lancet.* 2000; 355:1912.

5. Mai I, Kruger H, Budde K, et al. Hazardous pharmacokinetic interaction of Saint John's wort *(Hypericum perforatum)* with the immunosuppressant cyclosporin. *Int J Clin Pharmacol Ther.* 2000;38:500-502.

6. Dresser GK, Schwarz UI, Wilkinson GR, et al. St. John's wort induces intestinal and hepatic CYP3A4 and P-glycoprotein in healthy volunteers [abstract]. *Clin Pharmacol Ther.* 2001;69:P23.

7. Durr D, Stieger B, Kullak-Ublick GA, et al. St John's Wort induces intestinal P-glycoprotein/MDR1 and intestinal and hepatic CYP3A4. *Clin Pharmacol Ther.* 2000;68:598-604.

8. Sugimoto Ki K, Ohmori M, Tsuruoka S, et al. Different effects of St. John's Wort on the pharmacokinetics of simvastatin and pravastatin. *Clin Pharmacol Ther.* 2001;70:518-524.

9. Markowitz JS, De Vane CL, Boulton DW, et al. Effect of St. John's wort *(Hypericum perforatum)* on cytochrome P-450 2D6 and 3A4 activity in healthy volunteers. *Life Sci.* 2000;66:PL133-PL139.

10. Roby CA, Anderson GD, Kantor E, et al. St. John's wort: effect on CYP3A4 activity. *Clin Pharmacol Ther.* 2000;67:451-457.

11. Nebel A, Schneider BJ, Baker R, et al. Potential metabolic interaction between St. John's wort and theophylline [letter]. *Ann Pharmacother.* 1999;33:502.

12. Moore LB, Goodwin B, Jones SA, et al. St. John's wort induces hepatic drug metabolism through activation of the pregnane X receptor. *Proc Natl Acad Sci U S A.* 2000;97:7500-7502.

Digoxin—Foxglove

1. *The Review of Natural Products.* St. Louis, Mo: Facts and Comparisons; 1999: Digitalis monograph.
2. Clark RF, Selden BS, Curry SC. Digoxin-specific Fab fragments in the treatment of oleander toxicity in a canine model. *Ann Emerg Med.* 1991;20:1073-1077.

Digoxin—Ginseng
(Eleutherococcus senticosus/*Siberian Ginseng*)

1. McRae S. Elevated serum digoxin levels in a patient taking digoxin and Siberian ginseng. *CMAJ.* 1996;155:293-295.

Digoxin—Kyushin

1. Suga T. Chemistry and pharmacology of Chansu, Taisha. *Chin Med J (Engl).* 1973;suppl 10:762-773.
2. Fushimi R, Tachi J, Amino N, et al. Chinese medicine interfering with digoxin immunoassays [letter]. *Lancet.* 1989;1:339.

Digoxin—Licorice

1. Walker BR, Edwards CR. Licorice-induced hypertension and syndromes of apparent mineralocorticoid excess. *Endocrinol Metab Clin North Am.* 1994;23:359-377.
2. Epstein MT, Espiner EA, Donald RA, et al. Liquorice toxicity and the renin-angiotensin-aldosterone axis in man. *Br Med J.* 1977; 1:209-210.
3. Wash LK, Bernard JD. Licorice-induced pseudoaldosteronism. *Am J Hosp Pharm.* 1975;32:73-74.
4. de Klerk GJ, Nieuwenhuis MG, Beutler JJ. Hypokalaemia and hypertension associated with use of liquorice flavoured chewing gum. *BMJ.* 1997;314:731-732.
5. Corsi FM, Galgani S, Gasparini C, et al. Acute hypokalemic myopathy due to chronic licorice ingestion: report of a case. *Ital J Neurol Sci.* 1983;4:493-497.
6. Blachley JD, Knochel JP. Tobacco chewer's hypokalemia: licorice revisited. *N Engl J Med.* 1980;302:784-785.

Digoxin—Magnesium

1. Cohen L, Kitzes R. Magnesium sulfate and digitalis-toxic arrhythmias. *JAMA.* 1983;249:2808-2810.

2. Landauer JA. Magnesium deficiency and digitalis toxicity [letter]. *JAMA.* 1984;251:730.

3. Toffaletti J. Electrolytes, divalent cations, and blood gases (magnesium). *Anal Chem.* 1991;63:192R-194R.

4. Whang R, Oei TO, Watanabe A. Frequency of hypomagnesemia in hospitalized patients receiving digitalis. *Arch Intern Med.* 1985;145:655-656.

5. Brown DD, Juhl RP. Decreased bioavailability of digoxin due to antacids and kaolin-pectin. *N Engl J Med.* 1976;295:1034-1037.

6. D'Arcy PF, McElnay JC. Drug-antacid interactions: assessment of clinical importance. *Drug Intell Clin Pharm.* 1987;21:607-617.

7. McElnay JC, Harron DWG, D'Arcy PF, et al. Interaction of digoxin with antacid constituents [letter]. *Br Med J.* 1978;1:1554.

8. Greenblatt DJ, Duhme DW, Koch-Weser J, et al. Evaluation of digoxin bioavailability in single-dose studies. *N Engl J Med.* 1973;289:651-654.

Digoxin—St. John's Wort

1. Johne A, Brockmuller J, Bauer S, et al. Pharmacokinetic interaction of digoxin with an herbal extract from St. John's wort *(Hypericum perforatum). Clin Pharmacol Ther.* 1999;66:338-345.

2. Dresser GK, Schwarz UI, Wilkinson GR, et al. St. John's wort induces intestinal and hepatic CYP3A4 and P-glycoprotein in healthy volunteers [abstract]. *Clin Pharmacol Ther.* 2001;69:P23.

3. Durr D, Stieger B, Kullak-Ublick GA, et al. St. John's Wort induces intestinal P-glycoprotein/MDR1 and intestinal and hepatic CYP3A4. *Clin Pharmacol Ther.* 2000;68:598-604.

4. Kim RB, Wandel C, Leake B, et al. Interrelationship between substrates and inhibitors of human CYP3A and P-glycoprotein. *Pharm Res.* 1999;16:408-414.

Estrogen—Boron

1. Naghii MR, Samman S. The effect of boron supplementation on its urinary excretion and selected cardiovascular risk factors in healthy male subjects. *Biol Trace Elem Res.* 1997;56:273-286.

2. Nielsen FH, Hunt CD, Mullen LM, et al. Effect of dietary boron on mineral, estrogen, and testosterone metabolism in post-menopausal women. *FASEB J.* 1987;1:394-397.

Estrogen—Dong Quai

1. Wilbur P. The phyto-estrogen debate. *Eur J Herbal Med.* 1996; 2:20-26.

2. Hirata JD, Swiersz LM, Zell B, et al. Does dong quai have estrogenic effects in postmenopausal women? A double-blind, placebo controlled trial. *Fertil Steril.* 1997;68:981-986.

Estrogen—Ginseng (Panax ginseng)

1. Palmer BV, Montgomery AC, Monteiro JC. Gin Seng and mastalgia [letter]. *Br Med J.* 1978;1:1284.

2. Oura H, Hiai S, Nakashima S, et al. Stimulating effect of the roots of *Panax ginseng* C. A. Meyer on the incorporation of labeled precursors into rat liver RNA. *Chem Pharm Bull (Tokyo).* 1971;19: 453-459.

3. Greenspan EM. Ginseng and vaginal bleeding [letter]. *JAMA.* 1983;249:2018.

4. Hopkins MP, Androff L, Benninghoff AS. Ginseng face cream and unexplained vaginal bleeding. *Am J Obstet Gynecol.* 1988; 159:1121-1122.

5. Keane FM, Munn SE, du Vivier AW, et al. Analysis of Chinese herbal creams prescribed for dermatological conditions. *BMJ.* 1999;318:563-564.

Estrogen—Ipriflavone

1. Agnusdei D, Gennari C, Bufalino L. Prevention of early postmenopausal bone loss using low doses of conjugated estrogens and the non-hormonal, bone-active drug ipriflavone. *Osteoporos Int.* 1995;5:462-466.

2. Choi YK, Han IK, Yoon HK. Ipriflavone for the treatment of osteoporosis. *Osteoporos Int.* 1997;7(suppl 3):S174-S178.

3. de Aloysio D, Gambacciani M, Altieri P, et al. Bone density changes in postmenopausal women with the administration of ipriflavone alone or in association with low-dose ERT. *Gynecol Endocrinol.* 1997;11:289-293.

4. Gambacciani M, Ciaponi M, Cappagli B, et al. Effects of combined low dose of the isoflavone derivative ipriflavone and estrogen replacement on bone mineral density and metabolism in postmenopausal women. *Maturitas.* 1997;28:75-81.

5. Melis GB, Paoletti AM, Bartolini R, et al. Ipriflavone and low doses of estrogens in the prevention of bone mineral loss in climacterium. *Bone Miner.* 1992;19(suppl):S49-S56.

6. Nozaki M, Hashimoto K, Inoue Y, et al. Treatment of bone loss in oophorectomized women with a combination of ipriflavone and conjugated equine estrogen. *Int J Gynaecol Obstet.* 1998; 62:69-75.

7. Hanabayashi T, Imai A, Tamaya T. Effects of ipriflavone and estriol on postmenopausal osteoporotic changes. *Int J Gynaecol Obstet.* 1995;51:63-64.

8. Yamazaki I. Effect of ipriflavone on the response of uterus and thyroid to estrogen. *Life Sci.* 1986;38:757-764.

9. Petilli M, Fiorelli G, Benvenuti S, et al. Interactions between ipriflavone and the estrogen receptor. *Calcif Tissue Int.* 1995; 56:160-165.

10. Cecchini MG, Fleisch H, Muhibauer RC. Ipriflavone inhibits bone resorption in intact and ovariectomized rats. *Calcif Tissue Int.* 1997;61(suppl 1):S9-S11.

Estrogen—Resveratrol

1. Gehm BD, McAndrews JM, Chien PY, et al. Resveratrol, a polyphenolic compound found in grapes and wine, is an agonist for the estrogen receptor. *Proc Natl Acad Sci U S A.* 1997;94: 14138-14143.

Etoposide—St. John's Wort

1. Baker RK, Brandt TL, Siegel D, et al. Inhibition of human DNA topoisomerase II-alpha by the naphtha-di-anthrone, hypericin [abstract]. *Proc Annu Meet Am Assoc Cancer Res.* 1998;39:422.

2. Peebles KA, Baker RK, Kurz EU, et al. Catalytic inhibition of DNA topoisomerase II-alpha by hypericin, a naphthodianthrone from St. John's wort *(Hypericum perforatum). Biochem Pharmacol.* 2001;62:1059-1070.

3. Guengerich FP. Cytochrome P-450 3A4: regulation and role in drug metabolism. *Annu Rev Pharmacol Toxicol.* 1999;39:1-17.

Fexofenadine—Fruit Juice

1. Bailey DG, Dresser GK, Munoz C, et al. Reduction of fexofenadine bioavailability by fruit juices [abstract]. *Clin Pharmacol Ther.* 2001;69:P21.

Fluoroquinolones—Minerals

1. Minami R, Inotsume N, Nakano M, et al. Effect of milk on absorption of norfloxacin in healthy volunteers. *J Clin Pharmacol.* 1993;33:1238-1240.

2. Neuvonen PJ, Kivisto KT, Lehto P. Interference of dairy products with the absorption of ciprofloxacin. *Clin Pharmacol Ther.* 1991;50:498-502.

3. Lehto P, Kivisto KT. Different effects of products containing metal ions on the absorption of lomefloxacin. *Clin Pharmacol Ther.* 1994;56:477-482.

4. Dudley MN, Marchbanks CR, Flor SC, et al. The effect of food or milk on the absorption kinetics of ofloxacin. *Eur J Clin Pharmacol.* 1991;41:569-571.

5. Flor S, Guay DR, Opsahl JA, et al. Effects of magnesium-aluminum hydroxide and calcium carbonate antacids on bioavailability of ofloxacin. *Antimicrob Agents Chemother.* 1990;34:2436-2438.

6. Polk RE, Healy DP, Sahai J, et al. Effect of ferrous sulfate and multivitamins with zinc on absorption of ciprofloxacin in normal volunteers. *Antimicrob Agents Chemother.* 1989;33:1841-1844.

7. Kara M, Hasinoff BB, McKay DW, et al. Clinical and chemical interactions between iron preparations and ciprofloxacin. *Br J Clin Pharmacol.* 1991;31:257-261.

8. Campbell NR, Kara M, Hasinoff BB, et al. Norfloxacin interaction with antacids and minerals. *Br J Clin Pharmacol.* 1992;33:115-116.

9. Lehto P, Kivisto KT, Neuvonen PJ. The effect of ferrous sulphate on the absorption of norfloxacin, ciprofloxacin, and ofloxacin. *Br J Clin Pharmacol.* 1994;37:82-85.

10. Lomaestro BM, Bailie GR. Quinolone-cation interactions: a review. *DICP.* 1991;25:1249-1258.

11. Nix DE, Wilton JH, Ronald B, et al. Inhibition of norfloxacin absorption by antacids. *Antimicrob Agents Chemother.* 1990;34:432-435.

12. Grasela TH Jr, Schentag JJ, Sedman AJ, et al. Inhibition of enoxacin absorption by antacids or ranitidine. *Antimicrob Agents Chemother.* 1989;33:615-617.

13. Shimada J, Shiba K, Oguma T, et al. Effect of antacid on absorption of the quinolone lomefloxacin. *Antimicrob Agents Chemother.* 1992;36:1219-1224.

14. Teng R, Dogolo LC, Willavize SA, et al. Effect of Maalox and omeprazole on the bioavailability of trovafloxacin. *J Antimicrob Chemother.* 1997;39(suppl B):93-97.

15. Shiba K, Sakamoto M, Nakazawa Y, et al. Effects of antacid on absorption and excretion of new quinolones. *Drugs.* 1995;49 (suppl 2):360-361.

Folate—Aluminum Hydroxide

1. Oakley GP, Adams MJ, Dickinson CM. More folic acid for everyone, now. *J Nutr.* 1996;126:751S-755S.

2. Benn A, Swan CH, Cooke WT, et al. Effect of intraluminal pH on the absorption of pteroylmonoglutamic acid. *Br Med J.* 1971;1: 148-150.

3. Russell RM, Golner BB, Krasinski SD, et al. Effect of antacid and H2 receptor antagonists on the intestinal absorption of folic acid. *J Lab Clin Med.* 1988;112:458-463.

4. Stumm W, Morgan JJ, eds. *Aquatic Chemistry: An Introduction Emphasizing Chemical Equilibria in Natural Waters.* 2nd ed. New York, NY: Wiley; 1981:240.

Folate—Carbamazepine

1. Oakley GP, Adams MJ, Dickinson CM. More folic acid for everyone, now. *J Nutr.* 1996;126:751S-755S.

2. Ono H, Sakamoto A, Eguchi T, et al. Plasma total homocysteine concentrations in epileptic patients taking anticonvulsants. *Metabolism.* 1997;46:959-962.

3. Kishi T, Fujita N, Eguchi T, et al. Mechanism for reduction of serum folate by antiepileptic drugs during prolonged therapy. *J Neurol Sci.* 1997;145:109-112.

4. Reynolds EH. Mental effects of anticonvulsants, and folic acid metabolism. *Brain.* 1968;91:197-214.

5. Hendel J, Dam M, Gram L, et al. The effects of carbamazepine and valproate on folate metabolism in man. *Acta Neurol Scand.* 1984;69:226-231.

6. Isojarvi JI, Pakarinen AJ, Myllyla VV. Basic haematological parameters, serum gamma-glutamyl-transferase activity, and erythrocyte folate and serum vitamin B_{12} levels during carbamazepine and oxcarbazepine therapy. *Seizure.* 1997;6:207-211.

7. Reynolds EH, Milner G, Matthews DM, et al. Anticonvulsant therapy, megaloblastic haemopoiesis and folic acid metabolism. *Q J Med.* 1966;35:521-537.

8. Lewis DP, Van Dyke DC, Willhite LA, et al. Phenytoin-folic acid interaction. *Ann Pharmacother.* 1995;29:726-735.

9. Lewis DP, Van Dyke DC, Stumbo PJ, et al. Drug and environmental factors associated with adverse pregnancy outcomes. Part I: Antiepileptic drugs, contraceptives, smoking, and folate. *Ann Pharmacother.* 1998;32:802-817.

10. Biale Y, Lewenthal H. Effect of folic acid supplementation on congenital malformations due to anticonvulsive drugs. *Eur J Obstet Gynecol Reprod Biol.* 1984;18:211-216.

11. Cuskelly GJ, McNulty H, Scott JM. Fortification with low amounts of folic acid makes a significant difference in folate status in young women: implications for the prevention of neural tube defects. *Am J Clin Nutr.* 1999;70:234-239.

12. Berg MJ, Stumbo PJ, Chenard CA, et al. Folic acid improves phenytoin pharmacokinetics. *J Am Diet Assoc.* 1995;95:352-356.

Folate—Cimetidine

1. Oakley GP, Adams MJ, Dickinson CM. More folic acid for everyone, now. *J Nutr.* 1996;126:751S-755S.

2. Benn A, Swan CH, Cooke WT, et al. Effect of intraluminal pH on the absorption of pteroylmonoglutamic acid. *Br Med J.* 1971;1:148-150.

3. Russell RM, Golner BB, Krasinski SD, et al. Effect of antacid and H2 receptor antagonists on the intestinal absorption of folic acid. *J Lab Clin Med.* 1988;112:458-463.

Folate—Methotrexate

1. Jackson RC. Biological effects of folic acid antagonists with antineoplastic activity. *Pharmacol Ther.* 1984;25:61-82.

2. Omer A, Mowat AG. Nature of anaemia in rheumatoid arthritis. IX. Folate metabolism in patients with rheumatoid arthritis. *Ann Rheum Dis.* 1968;27:414-424.

3. van Ede AE, Laan RF, Rood MJ, et al. Effect of folic or folinic acid supplementation on the toxicity and efficacy of methotrexate in rheumatoid arthritis: a forty-eight week, multicenter, randomized, double-blind, placebo-controlled study. *Arthritis Rheum.* 2001;44:1515-1524.

4. Duhra P. Treatment of gastrointestinal symptoms associated with methotrexate therapy for psoriasis. *J Am Acad Dermatol.* 1993;28: 466-469.

5. Morgan SL, Baggott JE, Vaughn WH, et al. Supplementation with folic acid during methotrexate therapy for rheumatoid arthritis. A double-blind, placebo-controlled trial. *Ann Intern Med.* 1994;121:833-841.

6. Griffith SM, Fisher J, Clarke S, et al. Do patients with rheumatoid arthritis established on methotrexate and folic acid 5 mg daily need to continue folic acid supplements long term? *Rheumatology (Oxford).* 2000;39:1102-1109.

7. Hunt PG, Rose CD, McIlvain-Simpson G, et al. The effects of daily intake of folic acid on the efficacy of methotrexate therapy in children with juvenile rheumatoid arthritis. A controlled study. *J Rheumatol.* 1997;24:2230-2232.

Folate—NSAIDs

1. Oakley GP, Adams MJ, Dickinson CM. More folic acid for everyone, now. *J Nutr.* 1996;126:751S-755S.

2. Baum CL, Selhub J, Rosenberg IH. Antifolate actions of sulfasalazine on intact lymphocytes. *J Lab Clin Med.* 1981;97:779-784.

3. Baggott JE, Morgan SL, Taisun HA, et al. Inhibition of folate-dependent enzymes by non-steroidal anti-inflammatory drugs. *Biochem J.* 1992;282:197-202.

4. Lawrence VA, Loewenstein JE, Eichner ER. Aspirin and folate binding: in vivo and in vitro studies of serum binding and urinary excretion of endogenous folate. *J Lab Clin Med.* 1984;103:944-948.

5. Krogh Jensen M, Ekelund S, Svendsen L. Folate and homocysteine status and haemolysis in patients treated with sulphasalazine for arthritis. *Scand J Clin Lab Invest.* 1996;56:421-429.

6. Selhub J, Dhar GJ, Rosenberg IH. Inhibition of folate enzymes by sulfasalazine (Rapid Publication). *J Clin Invest.* 1978;61: 221-224.

Folate—Oral Contraceptives

1. Mooij PN, Thomas C, Doesburg WH, et al. Multivitamin supplementation in oral contraceptive users. *Contraception.* 1991;44: 277-288.

2. Steegers-Theunissen RP, Van Rossum JM, Steegers EA, et al. Sub-50 oral contraceptives affect folate kinetics. *Gynecol Obstet Invest.* 1993;36:230-233.

3. Green TJ, Houghton LA, Donovan U, et al. Oral contraceptives did not affect biochemical folate indexes and homocysteine concentrations in adolescent females. *J Am Diet Assoc.* 1998;98:49-55.

Folate—Phenytoin

1. Lewis DP, Van Dyke DC, Willhite LA, et al. Phenytoin-folic acid interaction. *Ann Pharmacother.* 1995;29:726-735.

2. Oakley GP, Adams MJ, Dickinson CM. More folic acid for everyone, now. *J Nutr.* 1996;126:751S-755S.

3. Ono H, Sakamoto A, Eguchi T, et al. Plasma total homocysteine concentrations in epileptic patients taking anticonvulsants. *Metabolism.* 1997;46:959-962.

4. Berg MJ, Stumbo PJ, Chenard CA, et al. Folic acid improves phenytoin pharmacokinetics. *J Am Diet Assoc.* 1995;95:352-356.

5. Kishi T, Fujita N, Eguchi T, et al. Mechanism for reduction of serum folate by antiepileptic drugs during prolonged therapy. *J Neurol Sci.* 1997;145:109-112.

6. Lewis DP, Van Dyke DC, Stumbo PJ, et al. Drug and environmental factors associated with adverse pregnancy outcomes. Part I: Antiepileptic drugs, contraceptives, smoking, and folate. *Ann Pharmacother.* 1998;32:802-817.

7. Biale Y, Lewenthal H. Effect of folic acid supplementation on congenital malformations due to anticonvulsive drugs. *Eur J Obstet Gynecol Reprod Biol.* 1984;18:211-216.

8. Cuskelly GJ, McNulty H, Scott JM. Fortification with low amounts of folic acid makes a significant difference in folate status in young women: implications for the prevention of neural tube defects. *Am J Clin Nutr.* 1999;70:234-239.

Folate—Triamterene

1. Oakley GP, Adams MJ, Dickinson CM. More folic acid for everyone, now. *J Nutr.* 1996;126:751S-755S.

2. Mason JB, Zimmerman J, Otradovec CL, et al. Chronic diuretic therapy with moderate doses of triamterene is not associated with folate deficiency. *J Lab Clin Med.* 1991;117:365-369.

3. Lieberman FL, Bateman JR. Megaloblastic anemia possibly induced by triamterene in patients with alcoholic cirrhosis. Two case reports. *Ann Intern Med.* 1968;68:168-173.

Folate—Trimethoprim/Sulfamethoxazole

1. Oakley GP, Adams MJ, Dickinson CM. More folic acid for everyone, now. *J Nutr.* 1996;126:751S-755S.

2. Kahn SB, Fein SA, Brodsky I. Effects of trimethoprim on folate metabolism in man. *Clin Pharmacol Ther.* 1968;9:550-560.

3. Vinnicombe HG, Derrick JP. Dihydropteroate synthase from *Streptococcus pneumoniae:* characterization of substrate binding order and sulfonamide inhibition. *Biochem Biophys Res Commun.* 1999;258:752-757.

Furosemide—Ginseng/Germanium

1. Becker BN, Greene J, Evanson J, et al. Ginseng-induced diuretic resistance [letter]. *JAMA.* 1996;276:606-607.

2. Sanai T, Okuda S, Onoyama K, et al. Germanium dioxide-induced nephropathy: a new type of renal disease. *Nephron.* 1990;54:53-60.

3. Takeuchi A, Yoshizawa N, Oshima S, et al. Nephrotoxicity of germanium compounds: report of a case and review of the literature. *Nephron.* 1992;60:436-442.

4. Yun TK. Experimental and epidemiological evidence of the cancer-preventive effects of *Panax ginseng* C.A. Meyer. *Nutr Rev.* 1996; 54(11 pt 2):S71-S81.

Furosemide—Gossypol

1. Liu GZ, Ch'iu-Hinton K, Cao JA, et al. Effects of K salt or a potassium blocker on gossypol-related hypokalemia. *Contraception.* 1988;37:111-117.

2. Qian SZ, Jing GW, Wu XY, et al. Gossypol related hypokalemia. Clinicopharmacologic studies. *Chin Med J (Engl).* 1980;93:477-482.

Glyburide—Chromium

1. Anderson RA, Cheng N, Bryden NA, et al. Elevated intakes of supplemental chromium improve glucose and insulin variables in individuals with type 2 diabetes. *Diabetes.* 1997;46:1786-1791.

2. Ravina A, Slezack L. Chromium in the treatment of clinical diabetes mellitus [translated from Hebrew]. *Harefuah.* 1993;125: 142-145.

3. Jovanovic L, Gutierrez M, Peterson CM. Chromium supplementation for women with gestational diabetes mellitus. *J Trace Elem Exp Med.* 1999;12:91-97.

4. Rabinowitz MB, Gonick HC, Levin SR, et al. Effects of chromium and yeast supplements on carbohydrate and lipid metabolism in diabetic men. *Diabetes Care.* 1983;6:319-327.

Glyburide—Ginseng
(Panax ginseng, Panax quinquefolius)

1. Sotaniemi EA, Haapakoski E, Rautio A. Ginseng therapy in non-insulin-dependent diabetic patients. *Diabetes Care.* 1995;18:1373-1375.

2. Vuksan V, Sievenpiper JL, Koo VY, et al. American ginseng (*Panax quinquefolius* L) reduces postprandial glycemia in nondiabetic subjects and subjects with type 2 diabetes mellitus. *Arch Intern Med.* 2000;160:1009-1013.

3. Vuksan V, Xu Z, Jenkins AL, et al. American ginseng (*Panax quinquefolium* L.) improves long term glycemic control in type 2 diabetes. Presented at 60th Scientific Sessions of the American Diabetes Association; June 9-13, 2000; San Antonio, Texas.

4. Konno C, Sugiyama K, Kano M, et al. Isolation and hypoglycaemic activity of panaxans A, B, C, D and E, glycans of *Panax ginseng* roots. *Planta Med.* 1984;50:434-436.

5. Konno C, Murakami M, Oshima Y, et al. Isolation and hypoglycemic activity of panaxans Q, R, S, T and U, glycans of *Panax ginseng* roots. *J Ethnopharmacol.* 1985;14:69-74.

6. Oshima Y, Konno C, Hikino H. Isolation and hypoglycemic activity of panaxans I, J, K, and L, glycans of *Panax ginseng* roots. *J Ethnopharmacol.* 1985;14:255-259.

7. Tomoda M, Shimada K, Konno C, et al. Partial structure of panaxan A, a hypoglycemic glycan of *Panax ginseng* roots. *Planta Med.* 1984;50:436-438.

8. Yokozawa T, Kobayashi T, Oura H, et al. Studies on the mechanism of the hypoglycemic activity of ginsenoside-Rb_2 in streptozotocin-diabetic rats. *Chem Pharm Bull (Tokyo)*. 1985; 33:869-872.

9. Ng TB, Li WW, Yeung HW. Effects of ginsenosides, lectins and *Momordica charantia* insulin-like peptide on corticosterone production by isolated rat adrenal cells. *J Ethnopharmacol*. 1987;21:21-29.

10. Lee YJ, Chung E, Lee KY, et al. Ginsenoside-Rg_1, one of the major active molecules from *Panax ginseng*, is a functional ligand of glucocorticoid receptor. *Mol Cell Endocrinol*. 1997;133: 135-140.

Glyburide—Vitamin E

1. Paolisso G, D'Amore A, Giugliano D, et al. Pharmacologic doses of vitamin E improve insulin action in healthy subjects and non-insulin-dependent diabetic patients. *Am J Clin Nutr*. 1993;57:650-656.

2. Paolisso G, D'Amore A, Galzerano D, et al. Daily vitamin E supplements improve metabolic control but not insulin secretion in elderly type II diabetic patients. *Diabetes Care*. 1993;16:1433-1437.

Haloperidol—Kava

1. Schelosky L, Raffauf C, Jendroska K, et al. Kava and dopamine antagonism [letter]. *J Neurol Neurosurg Psychiatry*. 1995;58:639-640.

Haloperidol—Phenylalanine

1. Mosnik DM, Spring B, Rogers K, et al. Tardive dyskinesia exacerbated after ingestion of phenylalanine by schizophrenic patients. *Neuropsychopharmacology*. 1997;16:136-146.

2. Gardos G, Cole JO, Matthews JD, et al. The acute effects of a loading dose of phenylalanine in unipolar depressed patients with and without tardive dyskinesia. *Neuropsychopharmacology*. 1992;6:241-247.

Heparin—Phosphatidylserine

1. van den Besselaar AM. Phosphatidylethanolamine and phosphatidylserine synergistically promote heparin's anticoagulant effect. *Blood Coagul Fibrinolysis*. 1995;6:239-244.

2. Palatini P, Viola G, Bigon E, et al. Pharmacokinetic characterization of phosphatidylserine liposomes in the rat. *Br J Pharmacol.* 1991;102:345-350.

Heparin—Vitamin C

1. Owen CA, Tyce GM, Flock EV, et al. Heparin-ascorbic acid antagonism. *Mayo Clin Proc.* 1970;45:140-145.

Ibuprofen—Feverfew

1. Collier HO, Butt NM, McDonald-Gibson WJ, et al. Extract of feverfew inhibits prostaglandin biosynthesis [letter]. *Lancet.* 1980;2:922-923.

2. Sumner H, Salan U, Knight DW, et al. Inhibition of 5-lipoxygenase and cyclo-oxygenase in leukocytes by feverfew. Involvement of sesquiterpene lactones and other components. *Biochem Pharmacol.* 1992;43:2313-2320.

3. Williams CA, Hoult JR, Harborne JB, et al. A biologically active lipophilic flavonol from *Tanacetum parthenium. Phytochemistry.* 1995;38:267-270.

Indinavir—St. John's Wort

1. Guengerich FP. Cytochrome P-450 3A4: regulation and role in drug metabolism. *Annu Rev Pharmacol Toxicol.* 1999;39:1-17.

2. Ernst E. Second thoughts about safety of St John's wort. *Lancet.* 1999;354:2014-2016.

3. Piscitelli SC, Burstein AH, Chaitt D, et al. Indinavir concentrations and St. John's wort [letter]. *Lancet.* 2000;355:547-548.

4. Markowitz JS, DeVane CL, Boulton DW, et al. Effect of St. John's wort *(Hypericum perforatum)* on cytochrome P-450 2D6 and 3A4 activity in healthy volunteers. *Life Sci.* 2000;66:PL133-PL139.

5. Roby CA, Anderson GD, Kantor E, et al. St John's Wort: effect on CYP3A4 activity. *Clin Pharmacol Ther.* 2000;67:451-457.

6. Nebel A, Schneider BJ, Baker R, et al. Potential metabolic interaction between St. John's wort and theophylline [letter]. *Ann Pharmacother.* 1999;33:502.

7. Moore LB, Goodwin B, Jones SA, et al. St. John's wort induces hepatic drug metabolism through activation of the pregnane X receptor. *Proc Natl Acad Sci U S A.* 2000;97:7500-7502.

8. Dresser GK, Schwarz UI, Wilkinson GR, et al. St. John's wort induces intestinal and hepatic CYP3A4 and P-glycoprotein in healthy volunteers [abstract]. *Clin Pharmacol Ther.* 2001;69:P23.

9. Durr D, Stieger B, Kullak-Ublick GA, et al. St. John's wort induces intestinal P-glycoprotein/MDR1 and intestinal and hepatic CYP3A4. *Clin Pharmacol Ther.* 2000;68:598-604.

10. Sugimoto Ki K, Ohmori M, Tsuruoka S, et al. Different effects of St. John's wort on the pharmacokinetics of simvastatin and pravastatin. *Clin Pharmacol Ther.* 2001;70:518-524.

11. de Maat MM, Hoetelmans RM, Mathot RA, et al. Drug interaction between St. John's wort and nevirapine [letter]. *AIDS.* 2001;15:420-421.

Insulin—Vanadium

1. Shamberger RJ. The insulin-like effects of vanadium. *J Adv Med.* 1996; 9:121-131.

2. Halberstam M, Cohen N, Shlimovich P, et al. Oral vanadyl sulfate improves insulin sensitivity in NIDDM but not in obese nondiabetic subjects. *Diabetes.* 1996;45:659-666.

3. Domingo JL. Vanadium: a review of the reproductive and developmental toxicity. *Reprod Toxicol.* 1996;10:175-182.

4. Domingo JL, Gomez M, Llobet JM, et al. Oral vanadium administration to streptozotocin-diabetic rats has marked negative side-effects which are independent of the form of vanadium used. *Toxicology.* 1991;66:279-287.

Iron—Calcium Carbonate

1. Dawson-Hughes B, Seligson FH, Hughes VA. Effects of calcium carbonate and hydroxyapatite on zinc and iron retention in postmenopausal women. *Am J Clin Nutr.* 1986;44:83-88.

2. Hallberg L, Brune M, Erlandsson M, et al. Calcium: effect of different amounts on nonheme- and heme-iron absorption in humans. *Am J Clin Nutr.* 1991;53:112-119.

3. Cook JD, Dassenko SA, Whittaker P. Calcium supplementation: effect on iron absorption. *Am J Clin Nutr.* 1991;53:106-111.

4. Sokoll LJ, Dawson-Hughes B. Calcium supplementation and plasma ferritin concentrations in premenopausal women. *Am J Clin Nutr.* 1992;56:1045-1048.

Iron—H₂ Antagonists

1. Champagne ET. Low gastric hydrochloric acid secretion and mineral bioavailability. *Adv Exp Med Biol.* 1989;249:173-184.

2. Sturniolo GC, Montino MC, Rossetto L, et al. Inhibition of gastric acid secretion reduces zinc absorption in man. *J Am Coll Nutr.* 1991;10:372-375.

3. Sandstead HH. Zinc nutrition in the United States. *Am J Clin Nutr.* 1973;26:1251-1260.

4. Goldenberg RL, Tamura T, Neggers Y, et al. The effect of zinc supplementation on pregnancy outcome. *JAMA.* 1995;274:463-468.

5. Prasad AS. Role of zinc in human health. *Bol Asoc Med P R.* 1991;83:558-560.

6. Prasad AS. Zinc deficiency in women, infants, and children. *J Am Coll Nutr.* 1996;15:113-120.

7. Stang J, Story MT, Harnack L, et al. Relationships between vitamin and mineral supplement use, dietary intake, and dietary adequacy among adolescents. *J Am Diet Assoc.* 2000;100:905-910.

Iron Salts—Beverage Teas

1. Blumenthal M, ed. *The Complete German Commission E Monographs, Therapeutic Guide to Herbal Medicines.* Boston, Mass: Integrative Medicine Communications; 1998:487-498.

2. Newall CA, Anderson LA, Phillipson JD. *Herbal Medicines: A Guide for Health-Care Professionals.* London, England: Pharmaceutical Press; 1996:286.

3. Chung KT, Wong TY, Wei CI, et al. Tannins and human health: a review. *Crit Rev Food Sci Nutr.* 1998;38:421-464.

4. Merhav H, Amitai Y, Palti H, et al. Tea drinking and microcytic anemia in infants. *Am J Clin Nutr.* 1985;41:1210-1213.

5. Pizarro F, Olivares M, Hertrampf E, et al. Factors which modify the nutritional state of iron: tannin content of herbal teas [in Spanish; English abstract]. *Arch Latinoam Nutr.* 1994;44:277-280.

Levodopa/Carbidopa—BCAAs

1. Robertson DR, Higginson I, Macklin BS, et al. The influence of protein containing meals on the pharmacokinetics of levodopa in healthy volunteers. *Br J Clin Pharmacol.* 1991;31:413-417.

Levodopa/Carbidopa—Iron

1. Campbell NR, Hasinoff BB. Iron supplements: a common cause of drug interactions. *Br J Clin Pharmacol.* 1991;31:251-255.

Lithium—Herbal Diuretics

1. Pyevich D, Bogenschutz MP. Herbal diuretics and lithium toxicity [letter]. *Am J Psychiatry.* 2001;158:1329.

Magnesium—Furosemide

1. al-Ghamdi SM, Cameron EC, Sutton RA. Magnesium deficiency: pathophysiologic and clinical overview. *Am J Kidney Dis.* 1994; 24:737-752.

2. Martin BJ, Milligan K. Diuretic-associated hypomagnesemia in the elderly. *Arch Intern Med.* 1987;147:1768-1771.

3. Dorup I. Magnesium and potassium deficiency. Its diagnosis, occurrence and treatment in diuretic therapy and its consequences for growth, protein synthesis and growth factors. *Acta Physiol Scand Suppl.* 1994;618:1-55.

4. Douban S, Brodsky MA, Whang DD, et al. Significance of magnesium in congestive heart failure. *Am Heart J.* 1996;132:664-671.

5. Whang R, Whang DD, Ryan MP. Refractory potassium repletion: a consequence of magnesium deficiency (review article). *Arch Intern Med.* 1992;152:40-45.

Magnesium—Oral Contraceptives

1. Seelig MS. Interrelationship of magnesium and estrogen in cardiovascular and bone disorders, eclampsia, migraine and premenstrual syndrome. *J Am Coll Nutr.* 1993;12:442-458.

2. Blum M, Kitai A, Ariel I, Shnirer M, et al. Effect of oral contraceptive on the magnesium level in the serum [translated from Hebrew]. *Harefuah.* 1991;3:363-364.

Magnesium—Potassium-Sparing Diuretics

1. Devane J, Ryan MP. The effects of amiloride and triamterene on urinary magnesium excretion in conscious saline-loaded rats. *Br J Pharmacol.* 1981;72:285-289.

2. al-Ghamdi SM, Cameron EC, Sutton RA. Magnesium deficiency: pathophysiologic and clinical overview. *Am J Kidney Dis.* 1994;24: 737-752.

3. Dorup I. Magnesium and potassium deficiency. Its diagnosis, occurrence and treatment in diuretic therapy and its consequences for growth, protein synthesis and growth factors. *Acta Physiol Scand Suppl.* 1994;618:1-55.

Manganese—Calcium Carbonate

1. Freeland-Graves JH; Lin PH. Plasma uptake of manganese as affected by oral loads of manganese, calcium, milk, phosphorous, copper, and zinc. *J Am Coll Nutr.* 1991;10:38-43.

2. Davidsson L, Cederblad A, Lonnerdal B, et al. The effect of individual dietary components on manganese absorption in humans. *Am J Clin Nutr.* 1991;54:1065-1070.

Methyldopa—Iron

1. Campbell N; Paddock V; Sundaram R. Alteration of methyldopa absorption, metabolism, and blood pressure control caused by ferrous sulfate and ferrous gluconate. *Clin Pharmacol Ther.* 1988;43:381-386.

2. Campbell NR, Hasinoff BB. Iron supplements: a common cause of drug interactions. *Br J Clin Pharmacol.* 1991;31:251-255.

Nefazodone—St. John's Wort

1. Muller WE, Rossol R. Effects of *Hypericum* extract on the expression of serotonin receptors. *J Geriatr Psychiatry Neurol.* 1994;7(suppl 1):S63-S64.

2. Teufel-Mayer R, Gleitz J. Effects of long-term administration of *Hypericum* extracts on the affinity and density of the central serotonergic 5-HT1 A and 5-HT2 A receptors. *Pharmacopsychiatry.* 1997;30(suppl 2):113-116.

3. Muller WE, Kasper S. *Hypericum* extract (Li 160) as a herbal antidepressant. *Pharmacopsychiatry.* 1997;30(suppl 2):71-134.

4. Muller WE, Singer A, Wonnemann M, et al. Hyperforin represents the neurotransmitter reuptake inhibiting constituent of *Hypericum* extract. *Pharmacopsychiatry.* 1998;31(suppl 1):16-21.

5. DeMott K. St. John's wort tied to serotonin syndrome. *Clin Psychiatry News.* 1998;26(3):28.

6. Ernst E. Second thoughts about safety of St. John's wort. *Lancet.* 1999;354:2014-2016.

7. Gordon JB. SSRIs and St. John's wort: possible toxicity? [letter]. *Am Fam Physician.* 1998;57:950, 953.

8. Lantz MS, Buchalter E, Giambanco V. St. John's wort and anti-depressant drug interactions in the elderly. *J Geriatr Psychiatry Neurol.* 1999;12:7-10.

9. Hernandez AF, Montero N, Pla A, et al. Fatal moclobemide overdose or death caused by serotonin syndrome? *J Food Prot.* 1995;40:128-130.

10. Callaway JC, Grob CS. Ayahuasca preparations and serotonin reuptake inhibitors: a potential combination for severe adverse interactions. *J Psychoactive Drugs.* 1998;30:367-369.

11. Biber A, Fischer H, Romer A, et al. Oral bioavailability of hyperforin from *Hypericum* extracts in rats and human volunteers. *Pharmacopsychiatry.* 1998;31(suppl 1):36-43.

Niacin—Isoniazid

1. Shibata K, Marugami M, Kondo T. In vivo inhibition of kynurenine aminotransferase activity by isonicotinic acid hydrazide in rats. *Biosci Biotechnol Biochem.* 1996;60:874-876.

2. DiLorenzo PA. Pellagra-like syndrome associated with isoniazid therapy. *Acta Derm Venereol.* 1967;47:318-322.

3. Ishii N, Nishihara Y. Pellagra encephalopathy among tuberculous patients: its relation to isoniazid therapy. *J Neurol.* 1985;48:628-634.

Nifedipine—Peppermint Oil

1. Blumenthal M, ed. *The Complete German Commission E Monographs, Therapeutic Guide to Herbal Medicines.* Boston, Mass: Integrative Medicine Communications; 1998:181-182.

2. Hawthorn M, Ferrante J, Luchowski E, et al. The actions of peppermint oil and menthol on calcium channel dependent processes in intestinal, neuronal, and cardiac preparations. *Aliment Pharmacol Ther.* 1988;2:101-118.

3. Taylor BA, Luscombe DK, Duthie HL. Inhibitory effect of peppermint oil on gastrointestinal smooth muscle [abstract]. *Gut.* 1983;24:A992.

Nitrofurantoin—Magnesium

1. Naggar VF, Khalil SA. Effect of magnesium trisilicate on nitrofurantoin absorption. *Clin Pharmacol Ther.* 1979;25:857-863.

2. Mannisto P. The effect of crystal size, gastric content and emptying rate on the absorption of nitrofurantoin in healthy human volunteers. *Int J Clin Pharmacol Biopharm.* 1978;16:223-228.

Nitroglycerin—N-Acetyl Cysteine

1. Ardissino D, Merlini PA, Savonitto S, et al. Effect of transdermal nitroglycerin or N-acetylcysteine, or both, in the long-term treatment of unstable angina pectoris. *J Am Coll Cardiol.* 1997;29:941-947.

2. Iversen HK. N-acetylcysteine enhances nitroglycerin-induced headache and cranial arterial responses. *Clin Pharmacol Ther.* 1992;52:125-133.

3. May DC, Popma JJ, Black WH. In vivo induction and reversal of nitroglycerin tolerance in human coronary arteries. *N Engl J Med.* 1987;317:805-809.

4. Ghio S, deServi S, Perotti R, et al. Different susceptibility to the development of nitroglycerin tolerance in the arterial and venous circulation in humans. Effects of N-acetylcysteine administration. *Circulation.* 1992;86:798-802.

5. Hogan JC, Lewis MJ, Henderson AH. Chronic administration of N-acetylcysteine fails to prevent nitrate tolerance in patients with stable angina pectoris. *Br J Clin Pharmacol.* 1990;30:573-577.

6. Hogan JC, Lewis MJ, Henderson AH. N-acetylcysteine fails to attenuate haemodynamic tolerance to glyceryl trinitrate in healthy volunteers. *Br J Clin Pharmacol.* 1989;28:421-426.

NSAIDs—Gossypol

1. Waller DP, Zaneveld LJ, Farnsworth NR. Gossypol: pharmacology and current status as a male contraceptive. *Econ Med Plant Res.* 1985;1:87-112.

2. Woerdenbag HJ. Gossypol. In: Smet PA, et al., eds. *Adverse Effects of Herbal Drugs.* Vol. 2. Berlin, Germany: Springer-Verlag; 1993:195-208.

Nutrients—Bile Acid Sequestrants

1. Hoppner K, Lampi B. Bioavailability of folate following ingestion of cholestyramine in the rat. *Int J Vitam Nutr Res.* 1991;61:130-134.

2. West RJ, Lloyd JK. The effect of cholestyramine on intestinal absorption. *Gut.* 1975;16:93-98.

Omeprazole—St. John's Wort

1. Gulick RM, McAuliffe V, Holden-Wiltse J, et al. Phase I studies of hypericin, the active compound in St. John's wort, as an antiretroviral agent in HIV-infected adults. AIDS Clinical Trials Group Protocols 150 and 258. *Ann Intern Med.* 1999;130:510-514.

2. Kako MD, Al-Sultan II, Saleem AN. Studies of sheep experimentally poisoned with *Hypericum perforatum. Vet Hum Toxicol.* 1993;35:298-300.

3. Mirossay A, Mirossay L, Tothova J, et al. Potentiation of hypericin and hypocrellin-induced phototoxicity by omeprazole. *Phytomedicine.* 1999;6:311-317.

Oral Contraceptives—Androstenedione

1. King DS, Sharp RL, Vukovich MD, et al. Effect of oral androstenedione on serum testosterone and adaptations to resistance training in young men: a randomized controlled trial. *JAMA.* 1999;281:2020-2028.

2. Leder BZ, Longcope C, Catlin DH, et al. Oral androstenedione administration and serum testosterone concentrations in young men. *JAMA.* 2000;283:779-782.

Oral Contraceptives—Licorice

1. Stewart PM, Wallace AM, Valentino R, et al. Mineralocorticoid activity of liquorice: 11-beta-hydroxysteroid dehydrogenase deficiency comes of age. *Lancet.* 1987;2:821-824.

2. Walker BR, Edwards CR. Licorice-induced hypertension and syndromes of apparent mineralocorticoid excess. *Endocrinol Metab Clin North Am.* 1994;23:359-377.

3. Wash LK, Bernard JD. Licorice-induced pseudoaldosteronism. *Am J Hosp Pharm.* 1975;32:73-74.

4. Bernardi M, D'Intino PE, Trevisani F, et al. Effects of prolonged ingestion of graded doses of licorice by healthy volunteers. *Life Sci.* 1994;55:863-872.

5. de Klerk GJ, Nieuwenhuis MG, Beutler JJ. Hypokalaemia and hypertension associated with use of liquorice flavoured chewing gum. *BMJ.* 1997;314:731-732.

Oral Contraceptives—Soy

1. Martini MC, Dancisak BB, Haggans CJ, et al. Effects of soy intake on sex hormone metabolism in premenopausal women. *Nutr Cancer.* 1999;34:133-139.

Oral Contraceptives—St. John's Wort

1. Guengerich FP. Cytochrome P-450 3A4: regulation and role in drug metabolism. *Annu Rev Pharmacol Toxicol.* 1999;39:1-17.

2. Diminished effect of birth control pill with concurrent use of SJW has led to unwanted pregnancy. http://www.mpa.se/. Accessed 10 June 2002.

3. Gorski JC, Hamman MA, Wang Z, et al. The effect of St. John's wort on the efficacy of oral contraception. American Society for Clinical Pharmacology and Therapeutics Annual Meeting, March 24-27, 2002, Atlanta, GA; abstract MPI-80.

Orally Administered Drugs—Psyllium

1. Perlman BB. Interaction between lithium salts and ispaghula husk [letter]. *Lancet.* 1990;335:416.

Paroxetine—St. John's Wort

1. Muller WE, Rossol R. Effects of *Hypericum* extract on the expression of serotonin receptors. *J Geriatr Psychiatry Neurol.* 1994; 7(suppl 1):S63-S64.

2. Teufel-Mayer R, Gleitz J. Effects of long-term administration of *Hypericum* extracts on the affinity and density of the central serotonergic 5-HT1 A and 5-HT2 A receptors. *Pharmacopsychiatry.* 1997;30(suppl 2):113-116.

3. Muller WE, Kasper S. *Hypericum* extract (Li 160) as a herbal antidepressant. *Pharmacopsychiatry.* 1997;30(suppl 2):71-134.

4. Muller WE, Singer A, Wonnemann M, et al. Hyperforin represents the neurotransmitter reuptake inhibiting constituent of *Hypericum* extract. *Pharmacopsychiatry.* 1998;31(suppl 1):16-21.

5. Gordon JB. SSRIs and St. John's wort: possible toxicity? [letter]. *Am Fam Physician.* 1998;57:950, 953.

6. DeMott K. St. John's wort tied to serotonin syndrome. *Clin Psychiatry News.* 1998;26(3):28.

7. Lantz MS, Buchalter E, Giambanco V. St. John's wort and antidepressant drug interactions in the elderly. *J Geriatr Psychiatry Neurol.* 1999;12:7-10.

8. Hernandez AF, Montero N, Pla A, et al. Fatal moclobemide overdose or death caused by serotonin syndrome? *J Food Prot.* 1995;40:128-130.

9. Callaway JC, Grob CS. Ayahuasca preparations and serotonin reuptake inhibitors: a potential combination for severe adverse interactions. *J Psychoactive Drugs.* 1998;30:367-369.

10. Biber A, Fischer H, Romer A, et al. Oral bioavailability of hyperforin from *Hypericum* extracts in rats and human volunteers. *Pharmacopsychiatry.* 1998;31(suppl 1):36-43.

Penicillamine—Iron

1. Osman MA, Patel RB, Schuna A, et al. Reduction in oral penicillamine absorption by food, antacid, and ferrous sulfate. *Clin Pharmacol Ther.* 1983;33:465-470.

Penicillamine—Magnesium

1. Osman MA, Patel RB, Schuna A, et al. Reduction in oral penicillamine absorption by food, antacid, and ferrous sulfate. *Clin Pharmacol Ther.* 1983;33:465-470.

Pentobarbital—Eucalyptol

1. Jori A, Bianchetti A, Prestini PE. Effect of essential oils on drug metabolism. *Biochem Pharmacol.* 1969;18:2081-2085.

Pentobarbital—Valerian

1. Capasso A, De Feo V, De Simone F, et al. Pharmacological effects of aqueous extract from *Valeriana adscendens. Phytother Res.* 1996;10:309-312.

Phenelzine—Ephedra

1. Portz BS, Faul KC, Pensoneau JA. Revised method for HPLC/UV determination and SPE cleanup of ephedra alkaloids in dietary products and herbal preparations. *Lab Inf Bull (Rockville, Md.).* 1996;(4053):1-18.

2. Blumenthal M, ed. *The Complete German Commission E Monographs, Therapeutic Guide to Herbal Medicines.* Boston, Mass: Integrative Medicine Communications; 1998:125-126, 477.

Phenelzine—Ginseng

1. Shader RI, Greenblatt DJ. Phenelzine and the dream machine— ramblings and reflections. *J Clin Psychopharmacol.* 1985;5:65.

2. Jones BD, Runikis AM. Interaction of ginseng with phenelzine [letter]. *J Clin Psychopharmacol.* 1987;7:201-202.

3. Oura H, Hiai S, Nakashima S, et al. Stimulating effect of the roots of *Panax ginseng* C. A. Meyer on the incorporation of labeled precursors into rat liver RNA. *Chem Pharm Bull (Tokyo).* 1971;19: 453-459.

4. Baldwin CA, Anderson LA, Phillipson JD. What pharmacists should know about ginseng. *Pharm J.* 1986;237:583-586.

Phenprocoumon—St. John's Wort

1. Maurer A, Johne A, Bauer S, et al. Interaction of St. John's wort extract with phenprocoumon [abstract]. *Eur J Clin Pharmacol.* 1999;55:A22.

2. Yue QY, Bergquist C, Gerden B. Safety of St. John's wort *(Hypericum perforatum)* [letter]. *Lancet.* 2000;355:576-577.

3. Kohl C, Steinkellner M. Prediction of pharmacokinetic drug/drug interactions from in vitro data: interactions of the nonsteroidal anti-inflammatory drug lornoxicam with oral anticoagulants. *Drug Metab Dispos.* 2000;28:161-168.

4. Guengerich FP. Cytochrome P-450 3A4: regulation and role in drug metabolism. *Annu Rev Pharmacol Toxicol.* 1999;39:1-17.

Phenytoin—Ginkgo

1. Wada K, Ishigaki S, Ueda K, et al. An antivitamin B6, 4'- methoxypyridoxine, from the seed of *Ginkgo biloba* L. *Chem Pharm Bull (Tokyo).* 1985;33:3555-3557.

2. Mizuno N, Kawakami K, Morita E. Competitive inhibition between 4'-substituted pyridoxine analogues and pyridoxal for pyridoxal kinase from mouse brain. *J Nutr Sci Vitaminol.* 1980;26:535-543.

3. Yagi M, Wada K, Sakata M, et al. Studies on the constituents of edible and medicinal plants. IV. Determination of 4-O-methylpyridoxine in serum of the patient with gin-nan food poisoning [in Japanese; English abstract]. *Yakugaku Zasshi.* 1993; 113:596-599.

4. Arenz A, Klein M, Fiehe K, et al. Occurrence of neurotoxic 4'-O-methylpyridoxine in *Ginkgo biloba* leaves, ginkgo medications and Japanese ginkgo food. *Planta Med.* 1996;62:548-551.

Phenytoin—Shankhapushpi

1. Dandekar UP, Chandra RS, Dalvi SS, et al. Analysis of a clinically important interaction between phenytoin and Shankhapushpi, an Ayurvedic preparation. *J Ethnopharmacol.* 1992;35:285-288.

Phosphorus—Aluminum Hydroxide

1. Spencer H, Kramer L. Antacid-induced calcium loss. *Arch Intern Med.* 1983;143:657-659.

2. Lotz M, Zisman E, Bartter FC. Evidence for a phosphorus-depletion syndrome in man. *N Engl J Med.* 1968;278:409-415.

3. Cooke N, Teitelbaum S, Avioli LV. Antacid-induced osteomalacia and nephrolithiasis. *Arch Intern Med.* 1978;138:1007-1009.

Piroxicam—St. John's Wort

1. Blumenthal M, ed. *The Complete German Commission E Monographs, Therapeutic Guide to Herbal Medicines.* Boston, Mass: Integrative Medicine Communications; 1998:215.

2. Roots I, Reum T, Brockmoller J, et al. Evaluation of photosensitization of the skin upon single- and multipose-dose intake of *Hypericum* extract [abstract]. *Phytomedicine.* 1996/1997;3(suppl 1):108.

3. Brockmoller J, Reum T, Bauer S, et al. Hypericin and pseudo-hypericin: pharmacokinetics and effects on photosensitivity in humans. *Pharmacopsychiatry.* 1997;30(suppl):94-101.

4. Gulick R, Lui H, Anderson R, et al. Human hypericism: a photosensitivity reaction to hypericin (St. John's wort) [abstract]. *Int Conf AIDS*. 1992;8:B90.

5. Kako MD, Al-Sultan II, Saleem AN. Studies of sheep experimentally poisoned with *Hypericum perforatum*. *Vet Hum Toxicol*. 1993;35:298-300.

6. Bombardelli E, Morazzoni P. *Hypericum perforatum*. *Fitoterapia*. 1995;66:43-68.

7. Kochevar IE, Morison WL, Lamm JL, et al. Possible mechanism of piroxicam-induced photosensitivity. *Arch Dermatol*. 1986;122:1283-1287.

8. Weigand DA. Piroxicam-induced photosensitivity [letter]. *J Am Acad Dermatol*. 1985;12:373-374.

9. Fernandez de Corres L, Diez JM, Audicana M, et al. Photodermatitis from plant derivatives in topical and oral medicaments. *Contact Dermatitis*. 1996;35:184-185.

10. Gould JW, Mercurio MG, Elmets CA. Cutaneous photosensitivity diseases induced by exogenous agents. *J Am Acad Dermatol*. 1995;33:551-573.

11. Harth Y, Rapoport M. Photosensitivity associated with antipsychotics, antidepressants and anxiolytics. *Drug Saf*. 1996;14:252-259.

12. Potter TS, Hashimoto K. Cutaneous photosensitivity to medications. *Compr Ther*. 1994;20:414-417.

13. Vassileva SG, Mateev G, Parish LC. Antimicrobial photosensitive reactions. *Arch Intern Med*. 1998;158:1993-2000.

Prednisolone—Licorice

1. Tamura Y, Nishikawa T, Yamada K, et al. Effects of glycyrrhetinic acid and its derivatives on delta-4-5-alpha- and 5-beta-reductase in rat liver. *Arzneimittelforschung*. 1979;29:647-649.

2. Monder C, Stewart PM, Lakshmi V, et al. Licorice inhibits corticosteroid 11-beta-dehydrogenase of rat kidney and liver: in vivo and in vitro studies. *Endocrinology*. 1989;125:1046-1053.

3. Chen MF, Shimada F, Kato H, et al. Effect of glycyrrhizin on the pharmacokinetics of prednisolone following low dosage of prednisolone hemisuccinate. *Endocrinol Jpn*. 1990;37:331-341.

4. Chen MF, Shimada F, Kato H, et al. Effect of oral administration of glycyrrhizin on the pharmacokinetics of prednisolone. *Endocrinol Jpn.* 1991;38:167-174.

5. Ojima M. The effects of glycyrrhizin preparations on patients with difficulty in release from steroid treatment. *Minophagen Med Rev Suppl.* 1987;17:120-125.

6. Kumagai A, Nanaboshi M, Asanuma Y, et al. Effects of glycyrrhizin on thymolytic and immunosupressive action of cortisone. *Endocrinol Jpn.* 1967;14:39-42.

7. Homma M, Oka K, Niitsuma T, et al. A novel 11-beta-hydroxysteroid dehydrogenase inhibitor contained in saiboku-to, a herbal remedy for steroid-dependent bronchial asthma. *J Pharm Pharmacol.* 1994;46:305-309.

Primidone—Nicotinamide

1. Bourgeois BF, Dodson WE, Ferrendelli JA. Interactions between primidone, carbamazepine, and nicotinamide. *Neurology.* 1982;32:1122-1126.

Procyclidine—Betel Nut

1. Taylor RF, Al-Jarad N, John LM, et al. Betel-nut chewing and asthma. *Lancet.* 1992;339:1134-1136.

2. Deahl M. Betel nut-induced extrapyramidal syndrome: an unusual drug interaction. *Mov Disord.* 1989;4:330-333.

3. Siegel RK. Herbal intoxication: psychoactive effects from herbal cigarettes, tea, and capsules. *JAMA.* 1976;236:473-476.

Propranolol—Black Pepper

1. Bano G, Raina RK, Zutshi U, et al. Effect of piperine on bioavailability and pharmacokinetics of propranolol and theophylline in healthy volunteers. *Eur J Clin Pharmacol.* 1991;41:615-617.

2. Bano G, Amla V, Raina RK, et al. The effect of piperine on pharmacokinetics of phenytoin in healthy volunteers. *Planta Med.* 1987;53:568-569.

3. Johri RK, Zutshi U. An Ayurvedic formulation 'trikatu' and its constituents. *J Ethnopharmacol.* 1992;37:85-91.

4. Atal CK, Dubey RK, Singh J. Biochemical basis of enhanced drug bioavailablility by piperine: evidence that piperine is a potent inhibitor of drug metabolism. *J Pharmacol Exp Ther.* 1985; 232:258-262.

5. Bhat BG, Chandrasekhara N. Interaction of piperine with rat liver microsomes. *Toxicology.* 1987;44:91-98.

Protease Inhibitors—Garlic

1. Piscitelli SC. Use of complementary medicines by patients with HIV: full sail into uncharted waters. *Medscape HIV/AIDS.* 2000;6(3).

2. Piscitelli SC, Burstein AH, Welden N, et al. The effect of garlic supplements on the pharmacokinetics of saquinavir. *Clin Infect Dis.* 2002;34:234-238.

SAMe—Levodopa/Carbidopa

1. Bottiglieri T, Hyland K, Reynolds EH. The clinical potential of ademetionine (S-Adenosylmethionine) in neurological disorders. *Drugs.* 1994;48:137-152.

2. Liu X, Lamango N, Charlton C. L-dopa depletes S-adeno-sylmethionine and increases S-adenosyl homocysteine: relationship to the wearing-off effects [abstract]. *Abstr Soc Neurosci.* 1998; 24:1469.

3. Charlton CG, Crowell B Jr. Striatal dopamine depletion, tremors, and hypokinesia following the intracranial injection of S-adenosylmethionine: a possible role of hypermethylation in parkinsonism. *Mol Chem Neuropathol.* 1995;26:269-284.

4. Carrieri PB, Indaco A, Gentile S, et al. S-adenosylmethionine treatment of depression in patients with Parkinson's disease: a double-blind, crossover study versus placebo. *Curr Ther Res.* 1990;48:154-160.

Simvastatin/Niacin Therapy—Antioxidants

1. Cheung MC, Zhao XQ, Chait A, et al. Antioxidant supplements block the response of HDL to simvastatin-niacin therapy in patients with coronary artery disease and low HDL. *Arterioscler Thromb Vasc Biol.* 2001;21:1320-1326.

Spironolactone—Licorice

1. Salassa RM, Mattox VR, Rosevear JW. Inhibition of the "mineralocorticoid" activity of licorice by spironolactone. *J Endocrinol Metab.* 1962;22:1156-1159.

2. Stewart PM, Wallace AM, Valentino R, et al. Mineralocorticoid activity of liquorice: 11-beta-hydroxysteroid dehydrogenase deficiency comes of age. *Lancet.* 1987;2:821-824.

3. Walker BR, Edwards CR. Licorice-induced hypertension and syndromes of apparent mineralocorticoid excess. *Endocrinol Metab Clin North Am.* 1994;23:359-377.

4. Wash LK, Bernard JD. Licorice-induced pseudoaldosteronism. *Am J Hosp Pharm.* 1975;32:73-74.

5. Bernardi M, D'Intino PE, Trevisani F, et al. Effects of prolonged ingestion of graded doses of licorice by healthy volunteers. *Life Sci.* 1994;55:863-872.

Statin Drugs—Niacin

1. Jacobson TA, Amorosa LF. Combination therapy with fluvastatin and niacin in hypercholesterolemia: a preliminary report on safety. *Am J Cardiol.* 1994;73:25D-29D.

2. Kashyap ML, Evans R, Simmons PD, et al. New combination niacin/statin formulation shows pronounced effects on major lipoproteins and is well tolerated [abstract]. *J Am Coll Cardiol.* 2000;35(suppl A):326.

3. Wolfe ML, Vartanian SF, Ross JL, et al. Safety and effectiveness of Niaspan when added sequentially to a statin for treatment of dyslipidemia. *Am J Cardiol.* 2001;87:476-479.

4. Wink J, Giacoppe G, King J. Effect of very-low-dose niacin on high-density lipoprotein in patients undergoing long-term statin therapy. *Am Heart J.* 2002;143:514-518.

Tamoxifen—Tangeretin

1. Bracke ME, Bruyneel EA, Vermeulen SJ, et al. Citrus flavonoid effect on tumor invasion and metastases. *Food Technol.* 1994;48:121-124. Cited by: Bracke ME, Depypere HT, Boterberg T, et al. Influence of tangeretin on tamoxifen's therapeutic benefit in mammary cancer. *J Natl Cancer Inst.* 1999;91:354-359.

2. Bracke ME, Depypere HT, Boterberg T, et al. Influence of tangeretin on tamoxifen's therapeutic benefit in mammary cancer. *J Natl Cancer Inst.* 1999;91:354-359.

Tetracyclines—Iron

1. Neuvonen PJ. Interactions with the absorption of tetracyclines. *Drugs.* 1976;11:45-54.

2. Campbell NR, Hasinoff BB. Iron supplements: a common cause of drug interactions. *Br J Clin Pharmacol.* 1991;31:251-255.

3. Heinrich HC, Oppitz KH, Gabbe EE. Inhibition of iron absorption in man by tetracycline [in German; English abstract]. *Klin Wochenschr.* 1974;52:493-498.

4. Andersson KE, Bratt L, Dencker H, et al. Inhibition of tetracycline absorption by zinc. *Eur J Clin Pharmacol.* 1976;10:59-62.

5. Mapp RK, McCarthy TJ. The effect of zinc sulphate and of bicitropeptide on tetracycline absorption. *S Afr Med J.* 1976;50:1829-1830.

Theophylline—Ipriflavone

1. Monostory K, Vereczkey L. The effect of ipriflavone and its manin metabolites on theophylline biotransformation. *Eur J Drug Metab Pharm.* 1996;21:61-66.

2. Monostory K, Vereczkey L, Levai F, et al. Ipriflavone as an inhibitor of human cytochrome P450 enzymes. *Br J Pharmacol.* 1998;123:605-610.

3. Takahashi J, Kawakatsu K, Wakayama T, et al. Elevation of serum theophylline levels by ipriflavone in a patient with chronic obstructive pulmonary disease [letter]. *Eur J Clin Pharmacol.* 1992; 43:207-208.

Theophylline—St. John's Wort

1. Nebel A, Schneider BJ, Baker R, et al. Potential metabolic interaction between St. John's wort and theophylline [letter]. *Ann Pharmacother.* 1999;33:502.

2. De Smet PA, Touw DJ. Safety of St. John's wort *(Hypericum perforatum)* [letter]. *Lancet.* 2000;355:575-576.

Thyroid Hormone—Calcium

1. Butner LE, Fulco PP, Feldman G. Calcium carbonate-induced hypothyroidism [letter]. *Ann Intern Med.* 2000;132:595.

2. Schneyer CR. Calcium carbonate and reduction of levothyroxine efficacy [letter]. *JAMA.* 1998;279:750.

3. Singh N, Singh PN, Hershman JM. Effect of calcium carbonate on the absorption of levothyroxine. *JAMA.* 2000;283:2822-2825.

Thyroid Hormone—Carnitine

1. Benvenga S, Lakshmanan M, Trimarchi F. Carnitine is a naturally occurring inhibitor of thyroid hormone nuclear uptake. *Thyroid.* 2000;10:1043-1050.

2. Benvenga S, Ruggeri RM, Russo A, et al. Usefulness of L-carnitine, a naturally occurring peripheral antagonist of thyroid hormone action, in iatrogenic hyperthyroidism: a randomized, double-blind, placebo-controlled clinical trial. *J Clin Endocrinol Metab.* 2001;86:3579-3594.

Thyroid Hormone—Iron

1. Campbell NR, Hasinoff BB, Stalts H, et al. Ferrous sulfate reduces thyroxine efficacy in patients with hypothyroidism. *Ann Intern Med.* 1992;117:1010-1013.

Thyroid Hormone—Soy

1. Jabbar MA, Larrea J, Shaw RA. Abnormal thyroid function tests in infants with congenital hypothyroidism: the influence of soy-based formula. *J Am Coll Nutr.* 1997;16:280-282.

2. Divi RL, Chang HC, Doerge DR. Anti-thyroid isoflavones from soybean: isolation, characterization, and mechanisms of action. *Biochem Pharmacol.* 1997;54:1087-1096.

3. Chorazy PA, Himelhoch S, Hopwood NJ, et al. Persistant hypothyroidism in an infant receiving a soy formula: a case report and review of the literature. *Pediatrics.* 1995;96:148-150.

Trimethoprim-Sulfamethoxazole—PABA

1. Vinnicombe HG, Derrick JP. Dihydropteroate synthase from *Streptococcus pneumoniae:* characterization of substrate binding order and sulfonamide inhibition. *Biochem Biophys Res Commun.* 1999;258:752-757.

2. Degowin RL, Eppes RB, Carson PE, et al. The effects of diaphenylsulfone (DDS) against chloroquine-resistant *Plasmodium falciparum*. *Bull World Health Organ*. 1966;34:671-681.

Trimethoprim-Sulfamethoxazole—Potassium

1. Alappan R, Perazella MA, Buller GK. Hyperkalemia in hospitalized patients treated with trimethoprim-sulfamethoxazole. *Ann Intern Med*. 1996;124:316-320.

Verapamil—Calcium

1. Hariman RJ, Mangiardi LM, McAllister RG Jr, et al. Reversal of the cardiovascular effects of verapamil by calcium and sodium: differences between electrophysiologic and hemodynamic responses. *Circulation*. 1979;59:797-804.

2. Watanabe Y, Nishimura M. Calcium—verapamil interaction on the AV node [letter]. *Int J Cardiol*. 1984;6:275-276.

3. Guadagnino V, Greengart A, Hollander G et al. Treatment of severe left ventricular dysfunction with calcium chloride in patients receiving verapamil. *J Clin Pharmacol*. 1987;27:407-409.

4. Salerno DM, Anderson B, Sharkey PJ, et al. Intravenous verapamil for treatment of multifocal atrial tachycardia with and without calcium pretreatment. *Ann Intern Med*. 1987;107:623-628.

5. Luscher TF, Noll G, Sturmer T, et al. Calcium gluconate in severe verapamil intoxication [letter]. *N Engl J Med*. 1994;330:718-720.

6. Orr GM, Bodansky HJ, Dymond DS, et al. Fatal verapamil overdose [letter]. *Lancet*. 1982;2:1218-1219.

7. Kuhn M, Schriger DL. Low-dose calcium pretreatment to prevent verapamil-induced hypotension. *Am Heart J*. 1992;124:231-232.

8. Midtbo K, Hals O. Can blood pressure reduction induced by slow calcium channel blockade (verapamil) be reversed by calcium infusion? *Pharmacol Toxicol*. 1987;60:330-332.

9. Bar-Or D, Gasiel Y. Calcium and calciferol antagonise effect of verapamil in atrial fibrillation. *Br Med J (Clin Res Ed)*. 1981;282:1585-1586.

Vitamin A—Valproic Acid

1. Nau H, Tzimas G, Mondry M, et al. Antiepileptic drugs alter endogenous retinoid concentrations: a possible mechanism of teratogenesis of anticonvulsant therapy. *Life Sci.* 1995;57:53-60.

Vitamin B₁ (Thiamine)—Loop Diuretics

1. Seligmann H, Halkin H, Rauchfleisch S, et al. Thiamine deficiency in patients with congestive heart failure receiving long-term furosemide therapy: a pilot study. *Am J Med.* 1991;91:151-155.

2. Shimon I, Almog S, Vered Z, et al. Improved left ventricular function after thiamine supplementation in patients with congestive heart failure receiving long-term furosemide therapy. *Am J Med.* 1995;98:485-490.

3. Brady JA, Rock CL, Horneffer MR. Thiamin status, diuretic medications, and the management of congestive heart failure. *J Am Diet Assoc.* 1995;95:541-544.

Vitamin B₂ (Riboflavin)—Oral Contraceptives

1. Larsson-Cohn U. Oral contraceptives and vitamins: a review. *Am J Obstet Gynecol.* 1975;121:84-90.

2. Webb JL. Nutritional effects of oral contraceptive use. *J Reprod Med.* 1980;25:150-156.

3. Wynn V. Vitamins and oral contraceptive use. *Lancet.* 1975;1:561-564.

Vitamin B₆ (Pyridoxine)—Isoniazid

1. Biehl JP, Vilter RW. Effect of isoniazid on vitamin B₆ metabolism; its possible significance in producing isoniazid neuritis. *Proc Soc Exp Biol Med.* 1954;85:389-392.

2. Heller CA, Friedman PA. Pyridoxine deficiency and peripheral neuropathy associated with long-term phenelzine therapy. *Am J Med.* 1983;75:887-888.

3. Snider DE Jr. Pyridoxine supplementation during isoniazid therapy. *Tubercle.* 1980;61:191-196.

4. Goldman AL, Braman SS. Isoniazid: a review with emphasis on adverse effects. *Chest.* 1972;62:71-77.

5. Vidrio H. Interaction with pyridoxal as a possible mechanism of hydralazine hypotension. *J Cardiovasc Pharmacol.* 1990;15:150-156.

Vitamin B₆ (Pyridoxine)—Levodopa

1. Leon AS, Spiegel HE, Thomas G, et al. Pyridoxine antagonism of levodopa in Parkinsonism. *JAMA.* 1971;218:1924-1927.

2. Yahr MD, Duvoisin RC. Pyridoxine and levodopa in the treatment of Parkinsonism. *JAMA.* 1972;220:861.

Vitamin B₆ (Pyridoxine)—Oral Contraceptives

1. Amatayakul K, Uttaravichai C, Singkamani R, et al. Vitamin metabolism and the effects of multivitamin supplementation in oral contraceptive users. *Contraception.* 1984;30:179-196.

2. van der Vange N, van den Berg H, Kloosterboer HJ, et al. Effects of seven low-dose combined contraceptives on vitamin B₆ status. *Contraception.* 1989;40:377-384.

3. Masse PG, van den Berg H, Duguay C, et al. Early effect of a low dose (30 µg) ethinyl estradiol-containing triphasil on vitamin B₆ status. A follow-up study on six menstrual cycles. *Int J Vitam Nutr Res.* 1996;66:46-54.

4. Kant AK, Block G. Dietary vitamin B₆ intake and food sources in the US population: NHANES II, 1976-1980. *Am J Clin Nutr.* 1990;52:707-716.

5. van der Wielen RP, de Groot LC, van Staveren WA. Dietary intake of water soluble vitamins in elderly people living in a Western society (1980-1993). *Nutr Res.* 1994;14:605-638.

6. Albertson AM, Tobelmann RC, Engstrom A, et al. Nutrient intakes of 2- to 10-year-old American children: 10-year trends. *J Am Diet Assoc.* 1992;92:1492-1496.

Vitamin B₆ (Pyridoxine)—Penicillamine

1. Rumsby PC, Shepherd DM. The effect of penicillamine on vitamin B₆ function in man. *Biochem Pharmacol.* 1981;30:3051-3053.

2. Kant AK, Block G. Dietary vitamin B-6 intake and food sources in the US population: NHANES II, 1976-1980. *Am J Clin Nutr.* 1990;52:707-716.

3. van der Wielen RP, de Groot LC, van Staveren WA. Dietary intake of water soluble vitamins in elderly people living in a Western society (1980-1993). *Nutr Res.* 1994;14:605-638.

4. Albertson AM, Tobelmann RC, Engstrom A, et al. Nutrient intakes of 2- to 10-year-old American children: 10-year trends. *J Am Diet Assoc.* 1992;92:1492-1496.

Vitamin B₆ (Pyridoxine)—Theophylline

1. Delport R, Ubbink JB, Vermaak WJH, et al. Theophylline increases pyridoxal kinase activity independently from vitamn B₆ nutritional status. *Res Commun Chem Pathol Pharmacol.* 1993;79: 325-333.

2. Shimizu T, Maeda S, Mochizuki H, et al. Theophylline attenuates circulating vitamin B₆ levels in children with asthma. *Pharmacology.* 1994;49:392-397.

3. Ubbink JB, Delport R, Bissbort S, et al. Relationship between vitamin B₆ status and elevated pyridoxal kinase levels induced by theophylline therapy in humans. *J Nutr.* 1990;120:1352-1359.

4. Bartel PR, Ubbink JB, Delport R, et al. Vitamin B-6 supplementation and theophylline-related effects in humans. *Am J Clin Nutr.* 1994;60:93-99.

5. Dakshinamurti K, Paulose CS, Viswanathan M. Vitamin B₆ and hypertension. *Ann N Y Acad Sci.* 1990;585:241-249.

6. Vestal RE, Eiriksson CE Jr, Musser B, et al. Effect of intravenous aminophylline on plasma levels of catecholamines and related cardiovascular and metabolic responses in man. *Circulation.* 1983;67: 162-171.

Vitamin B₁₂—Colchicine

1. Webb DI, Chodos RB, Mahar CQ, et al. Mechanism of vitamin B₁₂ malabsorption in patients receiving colchicine. *N Engl J Med.* 1968;279:845-850.

Vitamin B₁₂—H₂ Antagonists

1. Streeter AM, Goulston KJ, Bathur FA, et al. Cimetidine and malabsorption of cobalamin. *Dig Dis Sci.* 1982;27:13-16.

2. Salom IL, Silvis SE, Doscherholmen A. Effect of cimetidine on the absorption of vitamin B₁₂. *Scand J Gastroenterol.* 1982;17:129-131.

3. Belaiche J, Zittoun J, Marquet J, et al. Effect of ranitidine on secretion of gastric intrinsic factor and absorption of vitamin B₁₂ [translated from French]. *Gastroenterol Clin Biol.* 1983;7:381-384.

4. Saltzman JR, Kemp JA, Golner BB, et al. Effect of hypochlorhydria due to omeprazole treatment or atrophic gastritis on protein-bound vitamin B_{12} absorption. *J Am Coll Nutr.* 1994;13:584-591.

5. Marcuard SP, Albernaz L, Khazanie PG. Omeprazole therapy causes malabsorption of cyanocobalamin (vitamin B_{12}). *Ann Intern Med.* 1994;120:211-215.

Vitamin B_{12}—Metformin

1. Adams JF, Clark JS, Ireland JT, et al. Malabsorption of vitamin B_{12} and intrinsic factor secretion during biguanide therapy. *Diabetologia.* 1983;24:16-18.

2. Bauman WA, Shaw S, Jayatilleke E, et al. Increased intake of calcium reverses vitamin B_{12} malabsorption induced by metformin. *Diabetes Care.* 2000;23:1227-1231.

3. Schafer G. Some new aspects on the interaction of hypoglycemia-producing biguanides with biological membranes. *Biochem Pharmacol.* 1976;25:2015-2024.

4. Carmel R, Rosenberg AH, Lau KS, et al. Vitamin B_{12} uptake by human small bowel homogenate and its enhancement by intrinsic factor. *Gastroenterology.* 1969;56:548-555.

Vitamin B_{12}—Nitrous Oxide

1. Amos RJ, Amess JA, Hinds CJ, et al. Investigations into the effect of nitrous oxide anesthesia on folate metabolism in patient receiving intensive care. *Chemioterapia.* 1985;4:393-399.

2. Flippo TS, Holder WD Jr. Neurologic degeneration associated with nitrous oxide anesthesia in patients with vitamin B_{12} deficiency. *Arch Surg.* 1993;128:1391-1395.

3. Amos RJ, Amess JA, Hinds CJ, et al. Incidence and pathogenesis of acute megaloblastic bone-marrow change in patients receiving intensive care. *Lancet.* 1982;2:835-838.

4. Ermens AA, Refsum H, Rupreht J, et al. Monitoring cobalamin inactivation during nitrous oxide anesthesia by determination of homocysteine and folate in plasma and urine. *Clin Pharmacol Ther.* 1991;49:385-393.

5. Koblin DD, Tomerson BW, Waldman FM, et al. Effect of nitrous oxide on folate and vitamin B_{12} metabolism in patients. *Anesth Analg.* 1990;71:610-617.

6. Nunn JF, Chanarin I, Tanner AG, et al. Megaloblastic bone marrow changes after repeated nitrous oxide anaesthesia. Reversal with folinic acid. *Br J Anaesth*. 1986;58:1469-1470.

Vitamin B₁₂—Oral Contraceptives

1. Steegers-Theunissen RP, Van Rossum JM, Steegers EA, et al. Sub-50 oral contraceptives affect folate kinetics. *Gynecol Obstet Invest*. 1993;36:230-233.

2. Green TJ, Houghton LA, Donovan U, et al. Oral contraceptives did not affect biochemical folate indexes and homocysteine concentrations in adolescent females. *J Am Diet Assoc*. 1998;98:49-55.

3. Hjelt K, Brynskov J, Hippe E, et al. Oral contraceptives and the cobalamin (vitamin B₁₂) metabolism. *Acta Obstet Gynecol Scand*. 1985;64:59-63.

Vitamin C—Aspirin

1. Das N, Nebioglu S. Vitamin C aspirin interactions in laboratory animals. *J Clin Pharm Ther*. 1992;17:343-346.

2. Molloy TP, Wilson CW. Protein-binding of ascorbic acid. 2. Interaction with acetylsalicylic acid. *Int J Vitam Nutr Res*. 1980;50:387-392.

3. Coffey G, Wilson, CW. Letter: Ascorbic acid deficiency and aspirin-induced haematemesis. *Br Med J*. 1975;1:208.

Vitamin C—Oral Contraceptives

1. Rivers JM, Devine MM. Plasma ascorbic acid concentrations and oral contraceptives. *Am J Clin Nutr*. 1972;25:684-689.

2. Briggs M, Briggs M. Vitamin C requirements and oral contraceptives. *Nature*. 1972;238:277.

3. Larsson-Cohn U. Oral contraceptives and vitamins: a review. *Am J Obstet Gynecol*. 1975;121:84-90.

4. Webb JL. Nutritional effects of oral contraceptive use. *J Reprod Med*. 1980;25:150-156.

5. Wynn V. Vitamins and oral contraceptive use. *Lancet*. 1975;1:561-564.

Vitamin D—Cimetidine

1. Odes HS, Fraser GM, Krugliak P, et al. Effect of cimetidine on hepatic vitamin D metabolism in humans. *Digestion.* 1990;46:61-64.

2. [No authors listed]. Cimetidine inhibits the hepatic hydroxylation of vitamin D. *Nutr Rev.* 1985;43:184-185.

3. Bengoa JM, Bolt MJ, Rosenberg IH. Hepatic vitamin D 25-hydroxylase inhibition by cimetidine and isoniazid. *J Lab Clin Med.* 1984;104:546-552.

Vitamin D—Heparin

1. Aarskog D, Aksnes L, Markestad T, et al. Heparin-induced inhibition of 1,25-dihydroxyvitamin D formation. *Am J Obstet Gynecol.* 1984;148:1141-1142.

2. Haram K, Hervig T, Thordarson H, et al. Osteopenia caused by heparin treatment in pregnancy. *Acta Obstet Gynecol Scand.* 1993;72:674-675.

3. Wise PH, Hall AJ. Heparin-induced osteopenia in pregnancy. *Br Med J.* 1980;281:110-111.

Vitamin D—Isoniazid

1. Brodie MJ, Boobis AR, Hillyard CJ, et al. Effect of isoniazid on vitamin D metabolism and hepatic monooxygenase activity. *Clin Pharmacol Ther.* 1981;30:363-367.

2. Brodie MJ, Boobis AR, Dollery CT, et al. Rifampicin and vitamin D metabolism. *Clin Pharmacol Ther.* 1980;27:810-814.

3. Williams SE, Wardman AG, Taylor GA, et al. Long term study of the effect of rifampicin and isoniazid on vitamin D metabolism. *Tubercle.* 1985;66:49-54.

Vitamin D—Phenytoin

1. Brodie MJ, Boobis AR, Dollery CT, et al. Rifampicin and vitamin D metabolism. *Clin Pharmacol Ther.* 1980;27:810-814.

2. Jubiz W, Haussler MR, McCain TA, et al. Plasma 1,25-dihydroxyvitamin D levels in patients receiving anticonvulsant drugs. *J Clin Endocrinol Metab.* 1977;44:617-621.

3. Hahn TJ, Hendin BA, Scharp CR, et al. Effect of chronic anticonvulsant therapy on serum 25-hydroxycalciferol levels in adults. *N Engl J Med.* 1972;287:900-904.

4. Williams C, Netzloff M, Folkerts L, et al. Vitamin D metabolism and anticonvulsant therapy: effect of sunshine on incidence of osteomalacia. *South Med J.* 1984;77:834-836.

5. Tomita S, Ohnishi J, Nakano M, et al. The effects of anticonvulsant drugs on vitamin D_3–activating cytochrome P-450–linked monooxygenase systems. *J Steroid Biochem Mol Biol.* 1991;39: 479-485.

6. Weinstein RS, Bryce GF, Sappington LJ, et al. Decreased serum ionized calcium and normal vitamin D metabolite levels with anticonvulsant drug treatment. *J Clin Endocrinol Metab.* 1984;58: 1003-1009.

7. Wahl TO, Gobuty AH, Lukert BP. Long-term anticonvulsant therapy and intestinal calcium absorption. *Clin Pharmacol Ther.* 1981;30:506-512.

Vitamin D—Rifampin

1. Perry W, Erooga MA, Brown J, et al. Calcium metabolism during rifampicin and isoniazid therapy for tuberculosis. *J R Soc Med.* 1982;75:533-536.

2. Brodie MJ, Boobis AR, Dollery CT, et al. Rifampicin and vitamin D metabolism. *Clin Pharmacol Ther.* 1980;27:810-814.

Vitamin K—Amoxicillin

1. Cohen H, Scott SD, Mackie IJ, et al. The development of hypoprothrombinaemia following antibiotic therapy in malnourished patients with low serum vitamin K_1 levels. *Br J Haematol.* 1988;68:63-66.

2. Lipsky JJ. Nutritional sources of vitamin K. *Mayo Clin Proc.* 1994;69:462-466.

3. Conly J, Stein K. Reduction of vitamin K2 concentrations in human liver associated with the use of broad spectrum antimicrobials. *Clin Invest Med.* 1994;17:531-539.

4. Goss TF, Walawander CA, Grasela TH, et al. Prospective evaluation of risk factors for antibiotic-associated bleeding in critically ill patients. *Pharmacotherapy.* 1992;12:283-291.

5. Shearer MJ, Bechtold H, Andrassy K, et al. Mechanism of cephalosporin-induced hypoprothrombinemia: relation to cephalosporin side chain, vitamin K metabolism, and vitamin K status. *J Clin Pharmacol.* 1988;28:88-95.

Vitamin K—Cephalosporins

1. Cohen H, Scott SD, Mackie IJ, et al. The development of hypoprothrombinaemia following antibiotic therapy in malnourished patients with low serum vitamin K1 levels. *Br J Haematol.* 1988;68:63-66.

2. Shearer MJ, Bechtold H, Andrassy K, et al. Mechanism of cephalosporin-induced hypoprothrombinemia: relation to cephalosporin side chain, vitamin K metabolism, and vitamin K status. *J Clin Pharmacol.* 1988;28:88-95.

3. Goss TF, Walawander CA, Grasela TH, et al. Prospective evaluation of risk factors for antibiotic-associated bleeding in critically ill patients. *Pharmacotherapy.* 1992;12:283-291.

4. Allison PM, Mummah-Schendel LL, Kindberg CG, et al. Effects of a vitamin K-deficient diet and antibiotics in normal human volunteers. *J Lab Clin Med.* 1987;110:180-188.

5. Lipsky JJ. Nutritional sources of vitamin K. *Mayo Clin Proc.* 1994;69:462-466.

Vitamin K—Phenytoin

1. Cornelissen M, Steegers-Theunissen R, Kollee L, et al. Increased incidence of neonatal vitamin K deficiency resulting from maternal anticonvulsant therapy. *Am J Obstet Gynecol.* 1993;168(pt 1):923-928.

2. Cornelissen M, Steegers-Theunissen R, Kollee L, et al. Supplementation of vitamin K in pregnant women receiving anticonvulsant therapy prevents neonatal vitamin K deficiency. *Am J Obstet Gynecol.* 1993;168(pt 1):884-888.

3. Howe AM, Lipson AH, Sheffield LJ, et al. Prenatal exposure to phenytoin, facial development, and a possible role for vitamin K. *Am J Med Genet.* 1995;58:238-244.

Warfarin—Coenzyme Q$_{10}$

1. Combs AB, Porter TH, Folkers K. Anticoagulant activity of a naphtoquinone analog of vitamin K and an inhibitor of coenzyme Q10-enzyme systems. *Res Commun Chem Pathol Pharmacol.* 1976; 13:109-114.

2. Saupe J, Ronden JE, Soute BA, et al. Vitamin K-antagonistic effect of plastoquinone and ubiquinone derivatives in vitro. *FEBS Lett.* 1994;338:143-146.

3. Spigset O. Reduced effect of warfarin caused by ubidecarenone [letter]. *Lancet.* 1994;344:1372-1373.

Warfarin—Danshen

1. Chan TY. Interaction between warfarin and danshen *(Salvia miltiorrhiza). Ann Pharmacother.* 2001;35:501-504.

2. Lo AC, Chan K, Yeung JH, et al. The effects of Danshen *(Salvia miltiorrhiza)* on pharmacokinetics and pharmacodynamics of warfarin in rats. *Eur J Drug Metab Pharmacokinet.* 1992;17:257-262.

Warfarin—Dong Quai

1. Page RL 2nd, Lawrence JD. Potentiation of warfarin by dong quai. *Pharmacotherapy.* 1999;19:870-876.

2. Qiao S, Yao S, Wang Z. Coumarins of the root *Angelica dahurica. Planta Med.* 1996;62:584.

3. Tu JJ. Effects of radix *Angelicae sinensis* on hemorrheology in patients with acute ischemic stroke. *J Tradit Chin Med.* 1984;4: 225-228.

4. Ko FN, Wu TS, Liou MJ, et al. Inhibition of platelet thromboxane formation and phosphoinositides breakdown by osthole from *Angelica pubescens. Thromb Haemost.* 1989;62:996-999.

5. Lo AC, Chan K, Yeung JH, et al. Danggui *(Angelica sinensis)* affects the pharmacodynamics but not the pharmacokinetics of warfarin in rabbits. *Eur J Drug Metab Pharm.* 1995;20:55-60.

Warfarin—Feverfew

1. Heptinstall S, Groenewegen WA, Spangenberg P, et al. Extracts of feverfew may inhibit platelet behavior via neutralization of sulphydryl groups. *J Pharm Pharmacol.* 1987;39:459-465.

2. Makheja AN, Bailey JM. The active principle in feverfew [letter]. *Lancet*. 1981;2:1054.

3. Sumner H, Salan U, Knight DW, et al. Inhibition of 5-lipoxyge-nase and cyclo-oxygenase in leukocytes by feverfew. Involvement of sesquiterpene lactones and other components. *Biochem Pharmacol*. 1992;43:2313-2320.

4. Groenewegen WA, Heptinstall S. A comparison of the effects of an extract of feverfew and parthenolide, a component of feverfew, on human platelet activity in-vitro. *J Pharm Pharmacol*. 1990;42:553-557.

5. Biggs MJ, Johnson ES, Persaud NP, et al. Platelet aggregation in patients using feverfew for migraine [letter]. *Lancet*. 1982;2:776.

Warfarin—Garlic

1. Kiesewetter H, Jung F, Jung EM, et al. Effect of garlic on platelet aggregation in patients with increased risk of juvenile ischemic attack. *Eur J Clin Pharmacol*. 1993;45:333-336.

2. [No authors listed]. The effect of essential oil of garlic on hy-perlipemia and platelet aggregation—an analysis of 308 cases. Cooperative Group for Essential Oil of Garlic. *J Tradit Chin Med*. 1986;6:117-120.

3. Bordia A. Effect of garlic on human platelet aggregation in vitro. *Atherosclerosis*. 1978;30:355-360.

4. Srivastava KC. Evidence for the mechanism by which garlic in-hibits platelet aggregation. *Prostaglandins Leukot Med*. 1986;22:313-321.

5. Sharma CP, Nirmala NV. Effects of garlic extract and of three pure components isolated from it on human platelet aggregation, arachidonate metabolism, release reaction and platelet ultra-structure—comments [letter]. *Thromb Res*. 1985;37:489-490.

6. Harenberg J, Giese C, Zimmermann R. Effect of dried garlic on blood coagulation, fibrinolysis, platelet aggregation and serum cholesterol levels in patients with hyperlipoproteinemia. *Atherosclerosis*. 1988;74:247-249.

7. Mohammad SF, Woodward SC. Characterization of a potent in-hibitor of platelet aggregation and release reaction isolated from allium sativum (garlic). *Thromb Res*. 1986;44:793-806.

8. Apitz-Castro R, Escalante J, Vargas R, et al. Ajoene, the antiplatelet principle of garlic, synergistically potentiates the antiaggregatory action of prostacyclin, forskolin, indomethacin and dypiridamole on human platelets. *Thromb Res.* 1986;42:303-311.

9. Wagner H, Wierer M, Fessler B. Effects of garlic constituents on arachidonate metabolism. *Planta Med.* 1987;53:305-306.

10. Rose KD, Croissant PD, Parliament CF, et al. Spontaneous spinal epidural hematoma with associated platelet dysfunction from excessive garlic ingestion: a case report. *Neurosurgery.* 1990;26:880-882.

11. Sunter WH. Warfarin and garlic [letter]. *Pharmacol J.* 1991; 246:722.

Warfarin—Ginger

1. Backon J. Ginger: inhibition of thromboxane synthetase and stimulation of prostacyclin: relevance for medicine and psychiatry. *Med Hypotheses.* 1986;20:271-278.

2. Srivastava KC. Aqueous extracts of onion, garlic and ginger inhibit platelet aggregation and alter arachidonic acid metabolism. *Biomed Biochim Acta.* 1984;43:S335-S346.

3. Bordia A, Verma SK, Srivastava KC. Effect of ginger (*Zingiber officinale* rosc.) and fenugreek (*Trigonella foenumgraecum* L.) on blood lipids, blood sugar and platelet aggregation in patients with coronary artery disease. *Prostaglandins Leukot Essent Fatty Acids.* 1997;56:379-384.

4. Janssen PL, Meyboom S, van Staveren WA, et al. Consumption of ginger (*Zingiber officinale* roscoe) does not affect ex vivo platelet thromboxane production in humans. *Eur J Clin Nutr.* 1996; 50:772-774.

5. Lumb AB. Effect of dried ginger on human platelet function. *Thromb Haemost.* 1994;71:110-111.

Warfarin—Ginkgo

1. Rosenblatt M, Mindel J. Spontaneous hyphema associated with ingestion of *Ginkgo biloba* extract [letter]. *N Engl J Med.* 1997;336: 1108.

2. Vale S. Subarachnoid haemorrhage associated with *Ginkgo biloba* [letter]. *Lancet.* 1998;352:36.

3. Rowin J, Lewis SL. Spontaneous bilateral subdural hematomas associated with chronic *Ginkgo biloba* ingestion. *Neurology.* 1996;46:1775-1776.

4. Odawara M, Tamaoka A, Yamashita K. *Ginkgo biloba* [letter]. *Neurology.* 1997;48:789-790.

5. Chung KF, Dent G, McCusker M, et al. Effect of a ginkgolide mixture (BN 52063) in antagonising skin and platelet responses to platelet activating factor in man. *Lancet.* 1987;1:248-251.

Warfarin—Ginseng (Panax ginseng)

1. Janetzky K, Morreale AP. Probable interaction between warfarin and ginseng. *Am J Health Syst Pharm.* 1997;54:692-693.

2. Kuo SC, Teng CM, Lee JC, et al. Antiplatelet components in *Panax ginseng. Planta Med.* 1990;56:164-167.

3. Zhu M, Chan W, Ng S, et al. Possible influences of ginseng on the pharmacokinetics and pharmacodynamics of warfarin in rats. *J Pharm Pharmacol.* 1999;51:175-180.

Warfarin—Papaya Extract

1. Shaw D, Leon C, Kolev S, et al. Traditional remedies and food supplements: a 5-year toxicological study (1991-1995). *Drug Saf.* 1997;17:342-356.

2. Lambert JP, Cormier A. Potential interaction between warfarin and boldo-fenugreek. *Pharmacotherapy.* 2001;21:509-512.

Warfarin—Policosanol

1. Arruzazabala ML, Mas R, Molina V, et al. Effect of policosanol on platelet aggregation in type II hypercholesterolemic patients. *Int J Tissue React.* 1998;20:119-124.

2. Arruzazabala ML, Valdes S, Mas R, et al. Effect of policosanol successive dose increases on platelet aggregation in healthy volunteers. *Pharmacol Res.* 1996;34:181-185.

3. Arruzazabala ML, Valdes S, Mas R, et al. Comparative study of policosanol, aspirin and the combination therapy policosanol-aspirin on platelet aggregation in healthy volunteers. *Pharmacol Res.* 1997;36:293-297.

4. Cheema P, El-Mefty O, Jazieh AR. Intraoperative haemorrhage associated with the use of extract of saw palmetto herb: a case report and review of literature. *J Intern Med.* 2001;250:167-169.

Warfarin—Vinpocetine

1. Hitzenberger G, Sommer W, Grandt R. Influence of vinpocetine on warfarin-induced inhibition of coagulation. *Int J Clin Pharmacol Ther Toxicol.* 1990;28:323-328.

Warfarin—Vitamin A

1. Harris JE. Interaction of dietary factors with oral anticoagulants: review and applications. *J Am Diet Assoc.* 1995;95:580-584.

Warfarin—Vitamin C

1. Harris JE. Interaction of dietary factors with oral anticoagulants: review and applications. *J Am Diet Assoc.* 1995;95:580-584.

2. Rosenthal G. Interaction of ascorbic acid and warfarin [letter]. *JAMA.* 1971;215:1671.

3. Smith EC, Skalski RJ, Johnson GC, et al. Interaction of ascorbic acid and warfarin. *JAMA.* 1972;221:1166.

Warfarin—Vitamin E

1. Corrigan JJ Jr, Marcus FI. Coagulopathy associated with vitamin E ingestion. *JAMA.* 1974;230:1300-1301.

2. Schrogie JJ. Coagulopathy and fat-soluble vitamins [letter]. *JAMA.* 1975;232:19.

3. White JG, Rao GH, Gerrard JM. Effects of nitroblue tetrazolium and vitamin E on platelet ultrastructure, aggregation, and secretion. *Am J Pathol.* 1977;88:387-402.

4. Albanes D, Heinonen OP, Huttunen JK, et al. Effects of alpha-tocopherol and beta-carotene supplements on cancer incidence in the Alpha-Tocopherol Beta-Carotene Cancer Prevention Study. *Am J Clin Nutr.* 1995;62(suppl):1427S-1430S.

5. Kim JM, White RH. Effect of vitamin E on the anticoagulant response to warfarin. *Am J Cardiol.* 1996;77:545-546.

Warfarin—Vitamin K

1. Chow WH, Chow TC, Tse TM, et al. Anticoagulation instability with life-threatening complication after dietary modification. *Postgrad Med J.* 1990;66:855-857.

2. Pedersen FM, Hamberg O, Hess K, et al. The effect of dietary vitamin K on warfarin-induced anticoagulation. *J Intern Med.* 1991;229:517-520.

Zidovudine (AZT)—L-Carnitine

1. Dalakas MC, Leon-Monzon ME, Bernardini I, et al. Zidovudine-induced mitochondrial myopathy is associated with muscle carnitine deficiency and lipid storage. *Ann Neurol.* 1994;35:482-487.

2. Semino-Mora MC, Leon-Monzon ME, Dalakas MC. Effect of L-carnitine on the zidovudine-induced destruction of human myotubes. Part I: L-carnitine prevents the myotoxicity of AZT in vitro. *Lab Invest.* 1994;71:102-112.

3. Moretti S, Alesse E, Di Marzio L, et al. Effect of L-carnitine on human immunodeficiency virus-1 infection-associated apoptosis: a pilot study. *Blood.* 1998;91:3817-3824.

4. DeSimone C, Cifone MG, Alesse E, et al. Cell-associated ceramide in HIV-1-infected subjects [letter]. *AIDS.* 1996;10:675-676.

5. Kroemer G, Zamzami N, Susin SA. Mitochondrial control of apoptosis. *Immunol Today.* 1997;18:44-51.

Zinc—Amiloride

1. Reyes AJ, Olhaberry JV, Leary WP, et al. Urinary zinc excretion, diuretics, zinc deficiency and some side-effects of diuretics. *S Afr Med J.* 1983;64:936-941.

2. Wester PO. Urinary zinc excretion during treatment with different diuretics. *Acta Med Scand.* 1980;208:209-212.

3. Fosmire GJ. Zinc toxicity. *Am J Clin Nutr.* 1990;51:225-227.

4. Sandstead HH. Zinc nutrition in the United States. *Am J Clin Nutr.* 1973;26:1251-1260.

5. Prasad AS. Role of zinc in human health. *Bol Asoc Med P R.* 1991;83:558-560.

6. Prasad AS. Zinc deficiency in women, infants, and children. *J Am Coll Nutr.* 1996;15:113-120.

7. Goldenberg RL, Tamura T, Neggers Y, et al. The effect of zinc supplementation on pregnancy outcome. *JAMA.* 1995;274:463-468.

8. Stang J, Story MT, Harnack L, et al. Relationships between vitamin and mineral supplement use, dietary intake, and dietary adequacy among adolescents. *J Am Diet Assoc.* 2000;100:905-910.

Zinc—Calcium Carbonate

1. Argiratos V, Samman S. The effect of calcium carbonate and calcium citrate on the absorption of zinc in healthy female subjects. *Eur J Clin Nutr.* 1994;48:198-204.

2. Hwang SJ, Lai YH, Chen HC, et al. Comparisons of the effects of calcium carbonate and calcium acetate on zinc tolerance test in hemodialysis patients. *Am J Kidney Dis.* 1992;19:57-60.

3. Pecoud A, Donzel P, Schelling JL. Effect of foodstuffs on the absorption of zinc sulfate. *Clin Pharmacol Ther.* 1975;17:469-474.

4. Dawson-Hughes B, Seligson FH, Hughes VA. Effects of calcium carbonate and hydroxyapatite on zinc and iron retention in postmenopausal women. *Am J Clin Nutr.* 1986;44:83-88.

5. Spencer H, Kramer L, Norris C, et al. Effect of calcium and phosphorus on zinc metabolism in man. *Am J Clin Nutr.* 1984;40:1213-1218.

6. Crowther RS, Marriott C. Counter-ion binding to mucus glycoproteins. *J Pharm Pharmacol.* 1984;36:21-26.

Zinc—Captopril

1. Golik A, Zaidenstein R, Dishi V, et al. Effects of captopril and enalapril on zinc metabolism in hypertensive patients. *J Am Coll Nutr.* 1998;17:75-78.

2. Golik A, Modai D, Averbukh Z, et al. Zinc metabolism in patients treated with captopril versus enalapril. *Metabolism.* 1990;39:665-667.

Zinc—Hydrochlorothiazide

1. Reyes AJ, Leary WP, Lockett CJ, et al. Diuretics and zinc. *S Afr Med J.* 1982;62:373-375.

2. Reyes AJ, Olhaberry JV, Leary WP, et al. Urinary zinc excretion, diuretics, zinc deficiency and some side-effects of diuretics. *S Afr Med J.* 1983;64:936-941.

Zinc—Oral Contraceptives

1. Webb JL. Nutritional effects of oral contraceptive use. *J Reprod Med.* 1980;25:150-156.

2. Sandstead HH. Zinc nutrition in the United States. *Am J Clin Nutr.* 1973;26:1251-1260.

3. Prasad AS. Role of zinc in human health. *Bol Asoc Med P R.* 1991; 83:558-560.

4. Prasad AS. Zinc deficiency in women, infants, and children. *J Am Coll Nutr.* 1996;15:113-120.

5. Goldenberg RL, Tamura T, Neggers Y, et al. The effect of zinc supplementation on pregnancy outcome. *JAMA.* 1995;274: 463-468.

6. Stang J, Story MT, Harnack L, et al. Relationships between vitamin and mineral supplement use, dietary intake, and dietary adequacy among adolescents. *J Am Diet Assoc.* 2000;100:905-910.

Zinc—Zidovudine

1. Baum MK, Javier JJ, Mantero-Atienza E, et al. Zidovudine-associated adverse reactions in a longitudinal study of asymptomatic HIV-1-infected homosexual males. *J Acquir Immune Defic Syndr.* 1991;4:1218-1226.

2. Herzlich BC, Ranginwala M, Nawabi I, et al. Synergy of inhibition of DNA synthesis in human bone marrow by azidothymidine plus deficiency of folate and/or B_{12}? *Am J Hematol.* 1990;33: 177-183.

3. Mocchegiani E, Rivabene R, Santini MT. Benefit of oral zinc supplementation as an adjunct to zidovudine (AZT) therapy against opportunistic infections in AIDS. *Int J Immunopharmacol.* 1995;17:719-727.

4. Paltiel O, Falutz J, Veilleux M, et al. Clinical correlates of subnormal vitamin B_{12} levels in patients infected with the human immunodeficiency virus. *Am J Hematol.* 1995;49:318-322.

Zolpidem—5-HTP

1. Elko CJ, Burgess JL, Robertson WO. Zolpidem-associated hallucinations and serotonin reuptake inhibition: a possible interaction. *Clin Toxicol.* 1998;36:195-203.

INDEX